LECTURE N

CLINICAL (

Barry W.

MD, FRCP, DCH*
*Senior Lecturer in Medicine
University of Sheffield
Honorary Consultant Physician
Royal Hallamshire Hospital and
Weston Park Hospital, Sheffield*

J. David Bradshaw

MB, ChB, FRCR, DMRT
*Consultant Radiotherapist and Oncologist
Weston Park Hospital, Sheffield
Honorary Clinical Lecturer in Radiotherapy
and Oncology, University of Sheffield*

SECOND EDITION

BLACKWELL SCIENTIFIC PUBLICATIONS

OXFORD LONDON EDINBURGH

BOSTON PALO ALTO MELBOURNE

TO HELEN AND ELSA

First published 1981
Second Edition 1986

Set by Downdell Ltd, Oxford
Printed by Biddles Ltd, Guildford
and King's Lynn

DISTRIBUTORS

USA
  Blackwell Mosby Book Distributors
  11830 Westline Industrial Drive
  St Louis, Missouri 63141

Canada
  The C.V. Mosby Company
  5240 Finch Avenue East
  Scarborough, Ontario

Australia
  Blackwell Scientific Publications
  (Australia) Pty Ltd
  107 Barry Street
  Carlton, Victoria 3053

British Library
Cataloguing in Publication Data

Hancock, Barry W.
  Lecture notes on clinical
oncology.—2nd ed.
  1. Cancer
  I. Title   II. Bradshaw, J. David
  616.99′4   RC261

  ISBN 0-632-01548-9

Contents

Preface to Second Edition

Our thanks to colleagues who have pointed out errors and omissions in the first edition. The second edition has been updated to encompass recent advances in technology and therapy. An extra chapter on oncological emergencies has been included.

Barry W. Hancock
J. David Bradshaw

Preface to First Edition

This new book in the 'Lecture Notes' series is aimed at senior undergraduate students and recently qualified practitioners in all specialities; it is intended as an up-to-date guide to the theory and practice of all aspects of clinical oncology and should provide insight into the diverse nature of the subject, emphasising the multidisciplinary approach necessary for the successful management of the patient with cancer. We hope that our attempt to cover such a large field concisely will not contain too many omissions or dogmatisms. We are grateful to Professor J. Richmond, Dr F. E. Neal and Dr E. M. Pickering for helpful criticism and to the Department of Medical Illustration, Royal Hallamshire Hospital, Sheffield, for their help with many of the figures.

Chapter 1
Cancer Overview

Incidence and epidemiology

Impressions can be very misleading, and this is especially true in respect of the incidence of malignant disease. A worker in general practice might well regard the overall incidence as low; one in a general hospital is likely to regard it as higher; one in a specialist oncological hospital might get the impression that it is very common.

In fact, in the United Kingdom about three new cases are diagnosed each year for every 1000 of the population. One in every five persons born is likely to develop some form of the disease at some time during life. The average general practitioner will see seven new cases each year, but will see some types of malignancy very rarely. Cancer is not the commonest cause of death; the annual death rate from cardiac diseases is approximately three times that from malignant disease.

Cancer registration

With the development of cancer registration schemes, accurate estimations of the incidence of the disease in general and of its different types have become possible. It has become evident that overall the incidence has changed little over the past 50 years.

The registration of new cases on presentation provides a much more accurate estimation of incidence than do mortality statistics. Successfully treated malignant disease may not contribute to an individual's death, and therefore may not feature in the certified cause of death. Nevertheless, the incidence of death from the disease must rank high in the emotional reactions to the disease, of people in general.

Changing incidence of diseases

Since the beginning of the present century, there has been a steady reduction in the infant mortality rate, due in large part to improved neonatal care, and more recently to the availability of antibiotics. Whereas the principal causes of death in early life were infectious diseases, tuberculosis and other lung diseases, malignant disease now shows a relatively increased incidence in childhood.

Age and sex incidence of malignancy

The incidence of malignancy increases with age for most types of the disease. However, it is higher in the first five years of life than in the next two 5-year periods, principally due to leukaemia, to tumours of the central nervous system and to embryonal tumours.

In an increasing and ageing population the number of patients developing the disease will increase, even though the incidence at any age remains the same, and despite the fact that the chance of dying of the disease at any one age is gradually decreasing.

The overall incidence is the same in males and in females, but the relative rates vary with age. Below the age of ten years, it is higher in males than in females; over the period 20–60 years it is somewhat higher in females, especially in the period 35–50 years due to the relatively high incidence of malignancy of the breast and uterine cervix; over the age of 60 years, the incidence in males is markedly higher than that in females. Fig. 1.1 reflects approximately the overall incidence of the disease by age.

In western countries, the order of overall incidence of malignant disease for each sex and site is shown approximately in Table 1.1 and Fig. 1.2.

The predominating type of malignancy also varies with age. In children of both sexes up to the age of ten years, brain tumours and the leukaemias are commonest. In males, testicular tumours are commonest in the age

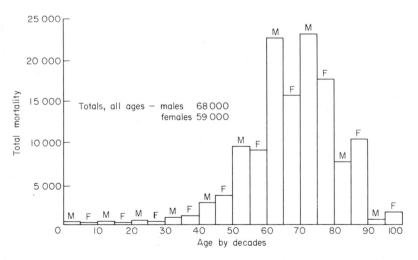

Fig. 1.1. Malignant disease; overall mortality by decades, England and Wales 1976. (Based on Government Statistical Service data from *Mortality Statistics—Cause*.)

Table 1.1. Incidence by site.

Males (%)	Females (%)
Bronchus (30)	Breast (25)
Digestive tract (20)	Digestive tract (20)
Urinary tract and prostate (15)	Uterus (10)
Skin (10)	Skin (10)
	Bronchus (5)

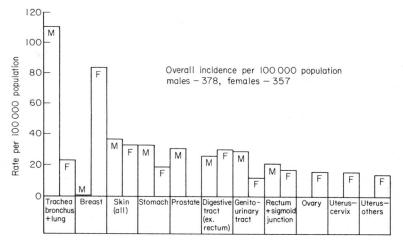

Fig. 1.2. Incidence of malignant disease by site. (Based on Trent Regional Health Authority data from *Radiotherapy Statistical Tables for 1977*.)

range 20–30 years, carcinoma of the bronchus in the age range 45–65 years, and adenocarcinoma of the prostate over the age of 70 years. In females, carcinomas of the breast and uterine cervix are commonest in the age range 25–65 years, and the predominance of carcinoma of the breast persists at all ages thereafter.

Geographical factors in incidence

The incidence of malignant disease can show marked variations between different countries and between different races. An outstanding example is the very low incidence of carcinoma of the uterine cervix in Jewish women. Other examples include the very high incidence of carcinoma of the postnasal space in the Chinese, the high incidence of malignancy of the

uterus in Indian women, of primary liver malignancy in South and West
Africans, of bladder malignancy in Egyptians, of stomach tumours in
Japanese and Scandinavians, and the very low incidence of breast
malignancy in the Japanese.

It is of great interest, however, to note that, in general, immigrant populations tend to assume the pattern of incidence appropriate to their adopted
country, suggesting that environmental factors have a major role in
aetiology.

Social factors in incidence (Table 1.2)

These environmental factors may be related to local geographical conditions, or to different life styles and habits. In females the age of marriage,
the number of pregnancies and the attitude to breast feeding may be relevant. To some extent, these factors may be determined by the degree of
economic development of the country, and the associated social and
economic status of the population. It is becoming increasingly evident that
environmental factors are responsible for many forms of malignant disease.

Industrial factors in incidence

As will be seen in more detail later the increased risk of workers in some
industries developing malignant disease is well recognised. As long ago as
1775, Percival Pott noted an association between carcinoma of the scrotal
skin and chimney sweeping as an occupation. Earlier this century, the
tendency to develop similar tumours in mule-spinners became evident,
this being related to the period when certain mineral oils were used to
lubricate the spindles of the mules.

More recently, an increased incidence of bladder carcinomas in workers
in the azo dye industry and in the rubber and cable industries has been

Table 1.2. Standardised mortality ratios by occupation, England and Wales
1970–72. (Based on Government Statistical Service data from *Social Trends*.)

Site	Professional and other		Inter-mediate		Skilled				Partly skilled		Unskilled	
					Non-manual		Manual					
	M	F	M	F	M	F	M	F	M	F	M	F
Trachea, bronchus and lung	53	73	68	82	84	89	118	118	123	125	143	134
Uterine cervix	—	<20	—	66	—	69	—	120	—	140	—	161
Breast	—	117	—	121	—	110	—	109	—	103	—	92
Prostate	91	—	89	—	99	—	115	—	106	—	115	—

recognised. Workers having prolonged contact with tar and pitch show a tendency to develop warty lesions in the exposed skin, and these can progress to become carcinomas. Prolonged contact with arsenical compounds can have similar effects.

Inhalation of dust containing chromates or dichromates can lead to lung malignancy; even more active is asbestos dust, which can result in tumours of the pleura (mesotheliomas) as well as of the bronchial mucosa. Long-term inhalation of benzol vapour can result in bone marrow changes ranging from anaemia and pancytopenia to leukaemia.

Prolonged exposure of the skin to strong sunlight will result in a higher than average incidence of keratotic lesions which have a marked tendency to undergo malignant change. This is seen, for example, in Indian tea planters and in Australian sheep farmers. The incidence of malignant melanoma of the skin increases with increasing exposure to ultraviolet light, natural or artificial.

Exposure over long periods to ionising radiations also can induce skin malignancies; this was seen particularly in early radiation workers, some of whom accumulated relatively large doses to the hands before the dangers were recognised.

All these forms of malignant disease are related to identifiable chemical carcinogens or to physical agents which can have carcinogenic effects. Once recognised, steps can be taken to limit or prevent exposure, or to introduce alternative non-carcinogenic agents in industry.

Mortality from malignancy

For many forms of the disease, mortality rates are showing a gradual fall; this is true particularly for malignancy of the stomach, uterus, bones and tongue. Malignancy of the pharynx is showing a fall in females but not in males. A rise in mortality is evident for malignancy of the ovary, pancreas, bladder, kidney and lung, and for the leukaemias and the lymphomas. The increasing mortality from carcinoma of the lung (bronchus) is most striking.

The overall mortality for males is higher than that for females. This is due to the higher incidence of malignancies of lower curability in males, especially bronchial and gastric carcinomas.

Changing mortality patterns therefore reflect firstly the changes in incidence and detection and secondly the effects of therapy on different tumours.

Aetiology

The precise cause of cancers is still unknown but it is likely that many, if not all, have a multifactorial aetiology. Genetic and environmental factors are important (Table 1.3).

Table 1.3. Factors related to the cause of cancer.

GENETIC

Familial predisposition to cancer
Chromosomal abnormality associated with increased incidence of cancer
Inherited syndromes associated with increased incidence of cancer
Histocompatibility antigen status predisposing to cancer

ENVIRONMENTAL

Irradiation
Chemicals
Viruses
Hormonal
Immunological
Chronic irritation

Genetic factors

There is evidence that individuals with certain genetic make-ups are more susceptible to cancer, though there is rarely a predictable mode of inheritance.

Familial predisposition

Some tumours occurring in children have a strong hereditary predisposition. One form of childhood retinoblastoma appears to be inherited as a dominant trait. Nephroblastoma, neuroblastoma, phaeocromocytoma and neurofibromatosis also have a strong familial element.

Chromosomal abnormality syndromes

In certain types of chromosomal abnormality disorders the incidence of neoplasia is increased. In Down's syndrome (trisomy 21) acute leukaemia is a well-known complication. This complication is also found in Klinefelter's syndrome (XXY), a condition in which breast carcinoma is also more common.

Associated inherited syndromes

Certain immunodeficiency syndromes are associated with an increased incidence of cancer. Ten per cent of patients with ataxia telangiectasia (an autosomal recessive disorder with telangiectasia, progressive ataxia and variable mixed immunodeficiency) and Wiskott–Aldrich syndrome (X-linked recessive immunodeficiency with eczema and thrombocytopenia) die of malignant disease, and the incidence may well be higher in patients with other variable immunodeficiency states. Lymphoreticular malignancy seems to be the commonest complication but the incidence of epithelial malignancy is also unexpectedly high.

Other 'non-immunodeficiency' disorders seem to predispose to cancer. Xeroderma pigmentosum, a skin condition with enhanced sun light sensitivity and increased incidence of skin and subcutaneous cancers, and polyposis coli predisposing to colonic carcinoma, are examples of these.

Histocompatibility antigen status

The histocompatibility antigen (human leucocyte antigen, HLA) system is a genetically determined single major transplantation antigen system, located within a region termed the major histocompatibility complex (MHC) on the 6th chromosome, which plays an important part in determining susceptibility and resistance to disease. Four of potentially many HLA gene loci have been identified—A, B, C and D (or D-related, DR). Particular HLA types are associated with malignancy, for example with Asiatic nasopharyngeal carcinoma (A2-Bw46) and long survivors with Hodgkin's disease (B8), acute lymphatic leukaemia (B2 and B9) and myelogenous leukaemia (B12).

An apparent increase of common cancers (such as breast, ovary and colon) is often seen in family groups; these could arise from some shared genetic characteristic, possibly HLA-mediated susceptibility, or equally from the action of similar environmental factors in a close-contact group or indeed from a combination of both.

Environmental factors

Irradiation

Ionising radiations have the capacity to displace electrons from atoms thus converting them to ions. They can therefore cause chemical changes within living cell molecules, the most important being the damage to the susceptible nuclear DNA with consequent changes in the structure and linkage of spiral strands. If these changes are severe enough cell death will result; less severe changes may cause the cells to become permanently altered in such a way as to escape normal control mechanisms—i.e. to become neoplastic.

Several examples of radiation induced tumours can be found. The high incidence of skin cancers in early X-ray workers, of lung cancer in the miners of radioactive ores, of bone tumours in girls who painted luminous watch dials (with radioactive radium), of thyroid cancer in people who survived the atomic bomb blasts or who had neck irradiation in childhood for some reason, and of leukaemia in patients with ankylosing spondylitis treated by radiotherapy, all suggest that radiation induces mutations in the genetic material of cells in the irradiated tissues.

Sunlight, by virtue of its ultraviolet irradiation, may over the years cause skin cancer in fair skinned people, presumably by damaging DNA in skin cells.

Chemicals

A list of the better known of the chemical carcinogens is given in Table 1.4. Many of them (probably more than 10%) are encountered during occupational exposure. Chemical carcinogens may be active in their primary form (direct acting) or may need to be modified in the body before becoming active (procarcinogens). Interference with nuclear DNA is again the main mechanism of oncogenesis.

Table 1.4. Chemical carcinogens and cancer.

OCCUPATIONAL EXPOSURE

Asbestos (lung)
Arsenic (skin, lung)
Chromium (lung)
Nickel (lung, paranasal sinuses)
PVC (liver)
Organic chemicals (lung, skin, bladder)
  petroleum fractions
  aromatic amines
  benzene

ENVIRONMENTAL AND FOOD

Aromatic hydrocarbons ⎫
Asbestos   ⎬ atmospheric (? lung)
Arsenic—drinking water (skin)
Aflatoxin—moulds (liver)
Preservatives (?)

SOCIAL CUSTOMS

Tobacco smoking (lung, oesophagus)

IATROGENIC

Arsenic (skin)
Cytotoxic drugs (various)
Immunosuppressive drugs (various)
Exogenous hormones (various)

Occupational. The most important occupational carcinogens are asbestos, arsenic, benzene, chromium, nickel and petroleum fractions, and it is important to remember that exposure to several of these chemicals can occur in one man's working lifetime with possible carcinogenesis of a number of tumours (e.g. lung carcinoma, mesothelioma, head and neck cancers). As has been seen, historically the soot induced scrotal carcinoma of chimney sweeps and the aniline dye induced bladder cancers achieved notoriety. More recently the effects of asbestos, particularly on the lung, of industrial mineral oils on the skin and of polyvinyl chloride (PVC) on the liver have provided the main debating points on chemical carcinogenesis.

Environmental. The importance of urban atmospheric pollution (e.g. with aromatic hydrocarbons and asbestos particles) in carcinogenesis is still uncertain. The roles of arsenic in drinking water of certain populations as a cause of skin cancer, and of aflatoxins from *Aspergillus flavis* in the staple foodstuffs of certain tropical peasants as a cause of liver cancer seem undeniable. There is also a causative association between pentose-rich fibres and lower gastrointestinal malignancy, and between poor nutrition and upper gastrointestinal cancer. In fact differences in diet probably account for more variation in the incidence of cancer than any other factor.

There are undoubtedly substances (e.g. nitrosamine) used as preservatives or colouring reagents in everyday foods, which if present in large enough quantities could be carcinogenic. The amounts present in food however are minute and the hazards which they present uncertain.

Social customs. Indisputably the main offender in this category is the habit of cigarette smoking—the carcinogenic effects of which are well known. The chewing of quids (beetle nuts, tobacco, burnt lime) is an important cause of oral cancer. Alcohol is thought to increase the incidence of mouth and throat cancer, particularly in smokers. It is estimated that tobacco has an aetiological role in 25–30% of all cancers.

Iatrogenic. Iatrogenic (doctor induced) chemical carcinogenesis is of uncertain importance but the effects of our new medications on the population may take years to evaluate. The carcinogenic problems seen at the present time are mainly related to the use of immunosuppressive and cytotoxic drugs in cancer, transplantation and autoimmune disease, and to the use of exogenous hormones (e.g. anabolic steroids and liver cancer, prenatal oestrogens and vaginal carcinoma).

Viruses

Several types of virus have been implicated in various animal tumours, both naturally occurring and experimentally induced. Perhaps the most important are the Polyoma and SV40 (Papova) viruses, which have been very useful in experimental cancer research, and the herpes type viruses, which have been incriminated in Marek's disease—a lymphoproliferative disorder of chickens.

There is little conclusive evidence of viral oncogenesis in man but circumstantial evidence suggests that infection may be an important cause in certain tumours. The occurrence of time–space clusters of patients with Hodgkin's disease and leukaemia is very suggestive of an infective aetiology. In carcinoma of the cervix an aetiological association with herpesvirus and/or human Papillomavirus type 16, is now apparent. In these conditions however, other environmental factors may be equally important. The hepatitis B virus also has a part to play in hepatoma.

No discussion of viral oncogenesis would be complete without mention of Burkitt's lymphoma. Patients with this type of lymphoma occur in clusters and invariably have antibodies to the Epstein–Barr virus; the virus has been isolated from cultured Burkitt's lymphoma cell lines. However the virus does in fact also cause infectious mononucleosis, a benign self-limiting infection, and it is difficult to see how the same virus could cause two such different disorders without some major host–virus adaptations. It now seems likely that chronic severe malaria depresses the host immunity in such a way as to allow continued infection with the virus and subsequent oncogenesis. The Epstein–Barr virus is also causally associated with nasopharyngeal carcinoma in the Chinese.

Another, albeit rare, neoplasm seen with viral infection is that caused by the human T cell leukaemia/lymphoma virus (HTLV) type I. It is also possible that this, or a similar virus, is involved in a T cell lymphoma of the skin (mycosis fungoides).

The acquired immune deficiency syndrome (AIDS) was first recognised as a new disease in 1981. Patients with this syndrome had persistent lymphadenopathy and were very susceptible to infections, as well as suffering from generalised ill health. These patients were found to have low helper/suppressor peripheral T cell ratios. The disease was noted to be more prevalent in homosexuals, drug abusers and recipients of blood products (particularly haemophiliacs), and patients were prone to develop rare opportunistic infections such as Pneumocystis carinii pneumonia. They also tended to develop malignancies such as Kaposi's sarcoma. This is normally an indolent malignancy, responsive to radio and/or chemotherapy; in AIDS however, it is very aggressive in its behaviour and may be rapidly lethal. It is now thought that a virus, HTLV type III, is causally associated with the development of AIDS. It is possible that some or all of the associated malignancies are caused by HTLV, or that the resulting immunosuppression allows other viruses (e.g. cytomegalovirus or Epstein–Barr virus) to become oncogenic.

Hormonal

Perhaps the most striking example of hormonal influence in cancer is in breast carcinoma. Some breast tumours are hormone responsive and this seems to correlate with the presence or absence of steroid receptor proteins in breast tissue cells. This has considerable therapeutic implications as we shall see later. It is likely that imbalance of endogenous hormones, rather than any direct oncogenic effects of these hormones, predisposes to cancer. Other examples of hormone dependent tumours are prostatic carcinoma and carcinoma of the body of the uterus.

Immunological

The role of immunology in the aetiology of tumours will be discussed more fully later. Suffice to say that one theory of oncogenesis is that potentially neoplastic cells are normally eradicated by a competent immuno-surveillance system; should this system become incompetent for any reasons (genetic or environmental) the cells escape control and proliferate, thus forming the cancer.

Chronic irritation

Cancers can arise at sites of chronic irritation, and in relation to scars, foreign bodies and chronic inflammation. Presumably cell damage at these sites gives rise to abnormal tissue differentiation. Oral cancer is probably the best example of this type of carcinogenesis—factors such as pipe smoking, ill-fitting dentures, poor dental hygiene and chronic infection (e.g. syphilis) are all recognised predisposing causes. In carcinoma of the vagina and cervix uteri there is an aetiological association with early coitus and/or poor genital hygiene. Certain chronic diseases also predispose to human cancer. Good examples of this are achlorhydria and pernicious anaemia and stomach cancer, Paterson-Kelly syndrome and post cricoid carcinoma, ulcerative colitis and colonic carcinoma, cirrhosis and hepatoma, Paget's disease and bone sarcoma, bilharzia and bladder cancer.

Oncogenes

A key problem in the fight against cancer is to find differences between normal and malignant cells. One such difference is now known to be located in small areas of the DNA of the genetic material (genome) of the cell. These are the so-called 'oncogenes' which are found in all normal cells (but in a repressed state). These cellular oncogenes (sometimes termed proto-oncogenes) closely resemble those found in viruses known to cause tumours in animals. Many RNA tumour viruses cause cancer in animals, and it seems that when such a virus infects a cell its RNA content is converted into double stranded DNA, which becomes integrated with the host chromosomal DNA so that the host cell starts to make viral type proteins which have the ability to transform cells. It is thought that cellular oncogenes in mammals are not merely the ineffective ancestors of viral oncogenes, but that they take a major part in the genesis of human cancer. They may well be involved in normal differentiation and growth control. It is likely that they are activated by carcinogens (e.g. radiation, chemicals and viruses) resulting in unrestrained cellular growth and tumour formation. Interestingly, some human oncogenes have been shown to be situated near the break-point of translocation chromosomal abnormalities—for example, an oncogene (the homologue of the Abelson murine leukaemia virus) is situated near the break-point of the translocation chromosome in chronic myeloid leukaemia (the Philadelphia chromosome, a 9.22 translocation). Translocation is also seen in Burkitt's lymphoma where an oncogene becomes fused with the immunoglobulin gene. It is possible that such translocations lead to amplification and expression of the cellular oncogene.

Summary

In summary, the underlying change in cancer is the abnormal differentiation of cells, probably by alteration of nuclear DNA, within the affected tissue. These cells escape normal growth-regulating mechanisms and proliferate to form a mass of tissue which grows beyond the normal confines of the tissue of origin. The initiating cause is likely to be multifactorial and many tumours are believed to arise because environmental factors (e.g. virus or chemical carcinogens) are operating in a host whose normal surveillance mechanisms are impaired by genetic predisposition.

It is probable that the two most important causative factors in cancer are diet and social customs (particularly tobacco smoking), accounting for at least two-thirds of cases. Other occupational and environmental factors are far less relevant.

Tumour biology

A tumour is formed when cells from a certain tissue escape the normal growth-regulating processes to extend beyond the normal confines of that tissue. The growth (neoplasm) can be benign or malignant. In the latter case the neoplasm has an ability to invade and destroy surrounding normal tissues and to spread to distant sites by a process known as metastasis; malignant tumours are generally termed cancers.

Tumour cells resemble normal cells in that they have the same structural features. Nuclear information is coded on the double stranded DNA (deoxyribonucleic acid) which is found in the chromosomes. The RNA (ribonucleic acid) is mainly concerned with protein synthesis within the cell cytoplasm. A special type of RNA (messenger RNA) conveys and translates the genetic information from the nucleus to the cytoplasmic RNA. The nucleotides are arranged in a chain-like pattern with sugar and phosphate groups, forming alternate links in the chain with nitrogenous bases (cytosine, thymine, adenine and guanine in DNA; cytosine, uracil, adenine and guanine in RNA) attached at each of the sugar units. The DNA complex is composed of two of these spiralling chains linked by hydrogen bonds across the nitrogen base units.

To undergo growth and division, the cell goes through a sequence of changes—the cell cycle.

The cell cycle (Fig. 1.3) is an ongoing phenomenon in which cells in cycle are in changeable equilibrium with cells in prolonged rest (G°). Cells in cycle go from an initial resting phase (G^1) through a synthetic phase (S) in which the cells' DNA content is doubled (tetraploidy), and after a further resting phase (G^2) undergo mitosis during which the parent cell splits into two identical daughter cells with identical DNA make-up. After this the daughter cells may recycle or go into prolonged rest (G°).

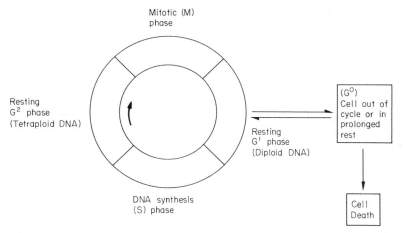

Fig. 1.3. Diagrammatic representation of the cell cycle.

Most of our information on cell cycling comes from animal and cell culture experiments and such data are difficult to translate *in vivo*. It is likely that human cells cycle over a period of 14–40 hours; the G^1 phase is the most variable in time interval and thus provides the difference between fast and slow dividing cell populations.

In the past it was commonly accepted that tumours increased in size because they cycled more rapidly; the numerous mitotic figures seen in tumour histology sections were held to support this view. Research has now shown that tumour cell cycling times are the same, or if anything longer, than those of normal cells. The explanation for tumour growth is in the imbalance between tumour cell formation and tumour cell loss (i.e. the failure to maintain a steady number of cells). New cells are added to the population at a greater rate than cells age and die, even though the cell loss from tumours is still considerable.

The other concept that people find difficult to understand is that usually the bigger the tumour the slower it grows (Fig. 1.4), i.e. its 'doubling time'—the time it takes the tumour to double its size—becomes longer because more and more cells go out of the cycle into a prolonged resting phase as the tumour grows in size. The cells left in cycle form the tumour growth fraction; this varies from 20–80% in different neoplasms.

Differences in the number of cells in the resting and growth compartments and in the rate of loss of cells from the tumour account for the variations in doubling times seen in different neoplasms; leukaemias have shorter doubling times than sarcomas, and carcinomas have the longest of all.

In their development cells need to specialise to function differently in particular tissues and organs. This process of differentiation is regulated by the genetic material coded on the DNA of the cell. It is likely that primitive cells are multipotent; they have the potential to differentiate into any of the

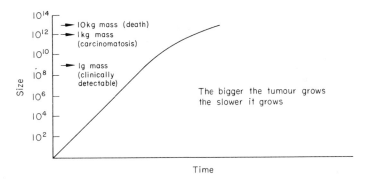

Fig. 1.4. Diagrammatic representation of tumour growth.

particular cell types found in that organism, but that this ability is normally repressed, except for the particular function required, by the action of the coded DNA.

Normal cells also seem to know their particular place in the organism in that they acknowledge positional signals. Cells from different tissues show the phenomenon of contact inhibition; they recognise and mix readily with cells of the same type but when confronted with cells of different types show antagonistic effects.

In the tumour cell differentiation is lost in varying degrees, presumably as a result of derepression or partial derepression of DNA genetic coding. Loss of function or inappropriate function may therefore result. The inability to recognise positional signals and the failure of contact inhibition in the tumour cells enables the cells to infiltrate normal tissues and to disseminate via blood and lymphatics to distant sites where they can survive in what should be alien territory.

There are approximately 10^{13} cells in the human body. In its lifetime a tumour will double its size 40 times to attain a size in excess of 1 kg; by that time there will be up to 10^{12} cells in the tumour. Unfortunately by the time it is clinically detected a tumour will be three-quarters of the way through its growth period and there must be the equivalent of at least a gram of tissue (10^9 cells) already present. In most patients more than 10^{10} cells are present at the time of clinical detection. It is only a short step further along the tumour's life history before 10^{12}–10^{13} cells are present and death of the patient occurs (Fig. 1.4).

Tumour pathology

Tumours are classified according to the tissue from which they originate. They may be benign or malignant, though it must be stressed there is considerable overlap and gradation between the two groups. The extent to which the tumour resembles its tissue of origin is noted in terms of degree of differentiation, so that a tumour resembling its parent tissue will be termed well differentiated; that showing little or no resemblance will be termed poorly differentiated or undifferentiated (anaplastic).

The six main sites of origin with the more common types of tumour are shown in Table 1.5.

Certain histological features help to distinguish tumour tissue from normal. The high mitotic activity seen in most malignant cells is more an index of the longer time spent by the cell in mitosis, with abnormal patterns of chromosomal division, than of mitotic rate since as we have already seen cancer cells do not divide faster than normal cells.

Table 1.5. Examples of benign and malignant neoplasms arising from various tissues.

	Neoplasm	
Tissue	Benign	Malignant
EPITHELIUM		
Squamous	Papilloma	Squamous carcinoma
Transitional	Papilloma	Transitional carcinoma
Glandular	Adenoma	Adenocarcinoma
CONNECTIVE TISSUE AND MUSCLES		
Fibrocyte	Fibroma	Fibrosarcoma
Fat cell	Lipoma	Liposarcoma
Muscle (smooth)	Leiomyoma	Leiomyosarcoma
Muscle (striated)	Rhabdomyoma	Rhabdomyosarcoma
Bone	Osteoma	Osteosarcoma
Vascular endothelium	Haemangioma	Haemangiosarcoma
Cartilage	Chondroma	Chondrosarcoma
HAEMPOIETIC AND LYMPHORETICULAR		
Erythrocyte	Polycythaemia vera	
Leucocyte		Leukaemia
Lymphoreticular cells	←———— Lymphomas ————→	
Plasma cell		Myeloma
NEURAL		
Neurocytes	Ganglioneuroma	Neuroblastoma
Glial cells	←——— Gliomas ———→	
Nerves	Neurilemmoma	Malignant neurilemmoma
	Neurofibroma	Neurofibrosarcoma
Meninges	Meningioma	Meningiosarcoma
EMBRYONAL AND GERMINAL		
Gonads		Seminoma
	←——— Teratomas ———→	
	Hydatidiform mole	Choriocarcinoma
Kidney		Nephroblastoma
Liver		Hepatoblastoma
Neural tissue		Neuroblastoma

The other histological features of malignant tumours have been noted already—dedifferentiation, invasion of adjacent tissues, microscopic evidence of metastases. Recognition of other more subtle microscopic changes requires the guidance of an experienced histopathologist.

Tumour immunology

It is now recognised that immunological reactions play a vital role in the modification and control of malignant disease.

Immunological response

The normal immunological response is extremely complex but is essentially a coordinated attack on foreign materials by two systems—phagocytic (circulating polymorphonuclear neutrophil leucocytes and reticuloendothelial macrophages) and lymphocytic (T and B lymphocytes). It is likely that the phagocytic system acts in the early stages of attack; in the inflammatory response target particles are phagocytosed, often in the presence of complement and opsonins, and are destroyed. If antigenic materials are produced at this stage then the lymphocytic response follows. T cells are concerned with the cellular immune response and with coordination of the total response to the antigen. They produce soluble mediator substances (lymphokines) which aid in the localisation of the immune reaction and in the destruction of the antigen. The humoral immune response is triggered by soluble antigens which have been processed by macrophages; after contact with these the B lymphocytes differentiate into plasma cells and produce immunoglobulins.

Using monoclonal antibodies (see p. 19) it is possible to define functional subsets of lymphocytes. It is now known that certain T cells may assist B cell antibody production (T helper/inducer cells); others modulate T helper cell function (the T suppressor cells) or are directly cytotoxic to target cells on contact. The helper/suppressor ratio (T4 : T8) in the blood is fairly constant (2 : 1) but may be reversed in immunodeficiency states. In addition certain cells (killer, K, or natural killer, NK) have antibody dependent cell-mediated cytotoxicity, and are believed to be of particular importance in defence against viral infections and in an immune surveillance role against cancer.

A number of low molecular weight products of macrophages and lymphocytes have been given the respective labels of monokines and lymphokines. One important monokine which activates lymphocytes is now called interleukin 1 (IL-1). There are many lymphokines, including interleukin 2 (IL-2), also called T cell growth factor, interferon (a major determinant of NK cell status), transfer factor, and various macrophage and leucocyte stimulating, chemotactic, migration and inhibition factors. Experimental and clinical research using these substances (particularly the interleukins and interferon) have been greatly helped by recent advances in molecular recombinant technology (see p. 71).

Immune surveillance

According to one theory of oncogenesis an organism's immunological system maintains a continuous surveillance over the development of abnormal and potentially neoplastic cells arising by a process of somatic mutation. If immunity is depressed for some reason there is theoretically a greater risk of developing cancer. This may be seen in practice; we have noted that patients with congenital immunological deficiency disease are at increased risk from cancers. Renal and cardiac transplant recipients on immunosuppressive therapy, and patients with Hodgkin's disease treated with cytotoxic chemotherapy, are also at increased risk of developing malignant disease. Further evidence of immunological protection against tumours comes from historical animal and human transplantation experiments. For example, homografts of cancer cells into normal people are rapidly rejected, whereas homografts into patients with advanced cancer are rejected slowly, if at all. Spontaneous tumour regression is also thought to result from improved host-immune response to the tumour and adds further support to the immunosurveillance theory. It is now thought likely however that this theory of oncogenesis is only part of a complex reaction of the host to the tumour.

We have also mentioned earlier that human leucocyte antigens (HLA) are a complex group of antigens present on tissue cell surfaces, and that certain significant associations between tissue antigens and malignancy have been observed. The immunological response genes are in close proximity to the histocompatibility genes and this is one possible explanation for the associations with cancer.

Tumour antigens

The evidence for the expression of specific antigens (neoantigens) on tumour cells is considerable; these antigens are sometimes called tumour-associated antigens and are believed to result from a reversion of the tumour cell to a primitive state with derepression and re-expression of the embryonic genes responsible for making these substances. It is however important to note that many of these oncofetal substances are present in small quantities in normal adult individuals. Many tumour antigens have been found, but only a few are of clinical importance. They are detected directly by radioimmunoassay or indirectly by assessing the sensitisation of the patient's lymphoid cells to the antigen. Carcinoembryonic antigen (CEA) is perhaps the best known. When its presence was first demonstrated it was thought to be specific for colonic carcinoma; subsequently, however, it was found to be present in many other tumours and indeed in all normal individuals, albeit at very low levels.

Alphafetoprotein (AFP) is also found in normal individuals and may be increased in pregnancy. Primary liver carcinoma is the most characteristic malignancy displaying elevation of AFP (more than 50% of patients), though raised levels are found in other tumours and particularly in teratomas.

Human chorionic gonadotrophins (HCG, βHCG) are of undoubted value in the monitoring of trophoblastic tumours (e.g. choriocarcinoma, teratoma) but can also be detected in the serum of patients with other tumours.

Other normal tissue substances (e.g. ferritin, an iron storage protein), may show biochemical and immunological changes in malignancy and can be used as tumour monitors.

Many authorities feel that the primary use of single or multiple tests for tumour antigens is in the follow-up of patients with tumours. Population screening is not a feasible proposition at the moment and the elevated levels of such antigens at the time of diagnosis may simply indicate the presence of extensive disease.

Monoclonal antibodies

Foreign antigens have specific regions to which a variety of immunoglobulins may bind. It is known that B lymphocytes are capable of producing immunoglobulins directed against each of these specific regions (monoclonal antibodies). Clones of lymphocytes can be stimulated to produce these specific antibodies. One way of doing this is to immunise laboratory animals, to extract the B lymphocytes from spleen tissue and to fuse these with a myeloma cell line. Clones of hybrid cells producing the wanted monoclonal antibody can be isolated and grown in suitable culture medium thus allowing an unlimited supply of antibody to be collected. Monoclonal antibodies, by their specificity, could theoretically recognise tumour cell antigens and thus certainly have a role in the diagnosis and localisation of tumours; they could be used as possible tumour markers and also, when labelled with fluorescein, in the identification of tumour cells in biopsies. They may also be of help in the localisation of tumours where the radio-labelled monoclonal antibody produced against the tumour tissue or marker substance localises the tumour *in vivo*, this being detected by gamma scanning (immunoscintography). There are also theoretical advantages in using monoclonal antibodies in the treatment of cancer, perhaps by conjugating the antibody with a cytotoxic substance thus targeting this on the tumour. Unfortunately, monoclonal antibodies do not themselves usually have a direct cytotoxic effect on cancer cells. However, one other use for them in therapy would be in the purging of autologous bone marrow of tumour cells before reintroduction into the patient (so-called bone marrow laundering).

Immunodeficiency

Immunodeficiency is another problem in patients with cancer, particularly in those with lymphoreticular malignancy or with disseminated disease. Quite often the presence of the cancer itself will be associated with immunosuppression; also the treatment given for the cancer (radiotherapy and chemotherapy) is immunosuppressive. Infections are therefore not uncommon in patients with widespread cancer undergoing therapy. The organisms responsible may cause only mild symptoms in normal individuals but can be severe or even fatal in the immunodepressed patient. Herpes zoster, *Candida albicans*, Varicella and common bacteria are the usual offenders, but more exotic infections (e.g. Aspergillus, Cryptococcus, Pneumocystis) can occur.

Growth of a tumour in its host will be more rapid if the tumour escapes the host's immunological control. This may happen as a result of the occurrence of immunological blocking factors. Excessive antibody production, deranged tumour cell antigen receptor sites and the formation of inappropriate antigen–antibody complexes can all interfere with the normally highly coordinated immunological attack. Not surprisingly the presence of blocking activity increases with increased tumour burden and diminishes when the tumour load is decreased.

The monitoring of immunological status can be helpful in the management and follow-up of patients with neoplastic disease, depressed immunity often being a feature of disseminated or relapsing cancer.

The role of immunotherapy in the treatment of cancer will be discussed in Chapter 5.

Effects of cancer

Cancers exert their effects in three main ways—by expansion and infiltration at their site of origin, by distant spread (metastasis) and by their remote (non-metastatic, paraneoplastic) effects (Fig. 1.5). Each particular type of neoplasm shows these effects in different degrees, e.g. sarcomas tend to infiltrate extensively locally before metastasising, certain differentiated thyroid tumours are notorious for metastasising early (the follicular type via bloodstream, the papillary type via lymphatics) and certain tumours, particularly bronchial carcinoma, can produce inappropriate hormones such as ACTH as a remote effect early in their development.

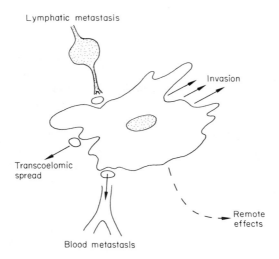

Lymphatic metastasis

Invasion

Transcoelomic spread

Remote effects

Blood metastasis

Fig. 1.5. The spread of cancer.

The paraneoplastic (non-metastatic, remote) effects of cancers are discussed fully in Chapter 16. They occur, but are sometimes not recognized, in many patients (more than 15%), particularly those with widespread disease. The commonest offending tumour is the bronchial carcinoma, particularly of the 'oat cell' type.

Cancer management—general comments

The ideal way to defeat cancer would be to prevent it. As we have indicated previously environmental factors are extremely important in the aetiology of tumours so that education about these factors and avoidance of them would possibly lower the incidence.

The large number of cells (10^9–10^{10}) present when the patient comes along with his cancer makes the problem of treatment enormous. Early detection by simple screening techniques if this were feasible would certainly help this problem.

The investigation and treatment of cancer involves the general practitioner, the hospital clinician, the radiologist, the pathologist and utilises many other laboratory services. A full history with examination will reveal the probable diagnosis in the majority of patients. Cancer must be confirmed, however, by biopsy and histological examination of appropriate tissues. Further investigations may be necessary to determine the extent of disease; these include haematological, biochemical and immunological blood investigations, radiology and radioisotope scanning.

In management the team approach is vital; the surgeon, radiotherapist and physician are all intensively involved. Any therapy must involve treating the tumour—if that is possible, and treating the patient—always. Attention to communication with the patient and his relatives will improve morale, allay fear and inspire confidence—all factors which make for better tolerance of what may be very uncomfortable treatment.

With curable tumours doctors can give, and patients can accept, traumatic therapy in the knowledge that a good result is possible. In the incurable lesion such physical and mental trauma is not justified; it is far better to help the symptoms with the minimum possible disturbance to the patient's remaining daily routine—the essence of cancer palliation.

Chapter 2
Investigation and Staging

Staging cancer

It has long been known that survival is longer for local than for widespread cancer. The concept of 'staging' has been applied to many tumours and individual staging procedures will be discussed in relation to specific cancers. However there may often be different staging procedures (clinical, surgical, radiological and pathological) for the same tumour, and this makes analysis and comparison of different treatment regimens and survival figures extremely difficult. The TNM system of classification was devised in an attempt to standardise staging by using basic principles applicable to all sites regardless of therapy. It enabled further information (histopathological, surgical) to be supplemented later to the initial clinical staging. The three components of the system are T (0-4), the extent of the primary tumour, N (0-4), the condition of regional lymph nodes and M (0-1), the absence or presence of distant metastases. Two categories of TNM classification are established, the pretreatment clinical, TNM, and post-surgical histopathological, p.TNM.

The TNM system has not been universally accepted, however, since the classifications for some tumours appear lengthy and sometimes cumbersome; it is nevertheless an attempt to rationalise many diverse staging procedures under one unifying concept.

Investigations

The staging of the patient depends on a full clinical and histopathological investigation. Some simple and baseline investigations are essential, and more complex procedures may also be necessary—dependent on the site and type of tumour and on the age and general condition of the patient. The young relatively fit patient with the potentially curable lesion will require much more extensive investigation than the elderly ill patient with an incurable solid tumour. Investigations are basically of four types:
1 tissue biopsy, 2 blood sampling, 3 radiological, 4 isotopic.

Tissue biopsy
The diagnosis of malignant disease must be established by the histological examination of a biopsy specimen from clinically involved tissue.

Blood sampling

Haematological investigations. A full peripheral blood count with examination of a blood film is mandatory in the patient with cancer. The erythrocyte sedimentation rate (ESR) is still one of the most important markers of disease activity, especially if monitored serially. Anaemia is common in malignancy. The blood film will give clues as to the nature of the anaemia, for example the microcytic hypochromic anaemia of blood loss, the normocytic normochromic anaemia of chronic disease, the leuco-erythroblastic picture of bone marrow replacement by tumour, and the macrocytic anaemia of folic acid deficiency.

The nature and differential count of peripheral white blood cells is also helpful. The presence of abnormal white cells in leukaemia or non-Hodgkin's lymphoma may suggest the diagnosis. Neutrophilia is sometimes a feature of widespread malignancy, as well as of bacterial infection. Neutropenia, lymphopenia and thrombocytopenia occur with widespread disease either as a toxic non-specific effect or as a result of bone marrow infiltration. Thrombocytosis is another non-specific effect of malignancy. Other haematological investigations which may be indicated are bone marrow examination as an aid to diagnosis of peripheral blood film abnormalities, serum ferritin to assess iron storage status, coagulation screening and platelet function studies in cases of thrombosis or bleeding, and red blood cell survival and autoantibody studies in cases of haemolysis.

Biochemical investigations. Blood samples should be taken for liver function tests (serum bilirubin, liver enzymes, alkaline phosphatase and proteins) and for urea, creatinine, calcium, uric acid and electrolyte assessment. Clinical assessment of hepatic involvement by cancer is difficult; hepatomegaly with deranged liver biochemistry does not mean pathological involvement by tumour, and conversely hepatic infiltration may be present in the absence of hepatomegaly and when the liver biochemistry is normal.

Immunological investigation. The importance of the immune response in cancer has been discussed (see Chapter 1). Assessment of immunological status in the patient with cancer is, however, optional since there is no conclusive proof that it relates to prognosis, and the tests involved are time consuming and sometimes difficult to interpret. Assessment may be important in patients with recurrent or serious problems with infection, or in those with tumours arising from 'immune' cells (leukaemia, lymphoma and myeloma). Various tests are possible; *in vivo* assessment of cellular immunity involves the use of active sensitisation with, for example, dinitrochlorobenzene or of skin testing with recall antigens. *In vitro* tests include the assessment of lymphocyte transformation with various mitogens, of leucocyte or macrophage inhibition responses to recall antigens, of T cell population study (E cell rosetting) and of various microcytotoxicity procedures. Humoral immunity assessment involves the measurement of serum immunoglobulins, of B cell populations (e.g. by immunofluorescent cell surface immunoglobulin labelling techniques) or of functional antibody formation, by natural antibody titres or after test immunisation. Functional subsets of immunologically active cells are now also defined using monoclonal antibodies.

Radiological investigations

Radiological examinations are of immense value in the assessment of patients with cancer, but should only be used where there is a good clinical indication. Having said this it is probably necessary to have a chest radiograph of most patients since this is still the best way of picking up metastatic disease; it will show up the presence of mediastinal/hilar lymph node involvement, of parenchymatous lung involvement by infiltration or by discrete or miliary deposits, and of pleuropericardial disease, usually effusions. Skeletal deposits (in ribs, clavicles, shoulder joints) may also be picked up on the chest X-ray.

Abnormalities detected on the standard chest X-ray may need to be followed with 'high kv' penetrating films or by tomographs to define their nature more clearly.

Skeletal radiographs may be indicated in tumours with a known tendency to metastasise to bone (such as breast, bronchus, prostate and myeloma), and often bone deposits are best detected by a screening survey (skeletal survey) of the axial skeleton. The primary indication for skeletal radiographs remains the presence of bone pain. Metastatic deposits, more often osteolytic than osteoblastic, are more frequently seen than primary bone tumours many of which have a characteristic X-ray appearance.

Gastrointestinal radiography includes the well established barium swallow, meal and follow-through and the barium enema examinations. Usually the investigations are undertaken to determine the underlying cause of specific symptoms or signs. For example, onset of dyspepsia or of changing bowel habit in the older patient may be the first sign of gastric or colonic carcinoma respectively, and unexplained iron deficiency anaemia may be the first sign of occult caecal carcinoma.

Adequate preparation for barium studies is vital if a high standard of examination is to be achieved. Particularly important is the bowel evacuation preparation needed for barium enema examination.

The techniques of gastroscopy, sigmoidoscopy and colonoscopy are complementary to the above barium studies.

Renal radiography usually involves intravenous pyelography (IVP). Kidney and bladder lesions and displacement or obstruction of the ureters can be visualised. In patients with impaired renal function high dose IVP may be necessary with late films (including renal tomograms) to detect delayed concentration and excretion of the contrast. Where renal impairment is thought to be due to obstruction retrograde pyelography may be indicated.

Bipedal lymphography still has a place in the investigation in malignant lymphoma and certain other tumours. The procedure involves the isolation of lymphatic vessels, on the dorsal surfaces of both feet, identified by the uptake of a marker dye injected into the skin above the toes. The lymphatic channel can be cannulated after cut-down and contrast (usually ultrafluid Lipiodol) is injected. The contrast is then visualised, by a series of X-rays, ascending the lymphatics of the leg and entering the lower abdominal lymph nodes. Twenty-four hour X-rays allow the visualisation of iliac and para-aortic nodes. The oily contrast remains in the nodes for many months.

The procedure has two basic aims: **1** to detect pelvic and abdominal lymph node involvement by the tumour, **2** in follow-up, to assess the success of therapy or the presence of tumour recurrence.

The lymph nodes in malignant lymphoma have the appearance of being large and foamy. With other tumours the lymph nodes may be enlarged but they more often show discrete filling defects. In all tumours complete replacement of lymph nodes will mean that they are not visualised on lymphography and this may be associated with lymphatic obstruction.

There is considerable overlap of the lymphographic appearances of various malignant tumours and of other diseases (e.g. sarcoidosis, infections, collagen-vascular diseases) and findings must be taken in conjunction with clinical assessment.

Complications of lymphography are uncommon (less than 1% in experienced hands). Allergic reactions to marker dye or contrast are usually transient with mild pyrexia or flu-like symptoms, but severe anaphylaxis can occur. Lipiodol, being an oily medium, embolises to the lungs and can cause minor pulmonary function abnormalities, mainly reduced gaseous diffusion; this becomes important in the patient with low respiratory reserve (e.g. chronic lung or heart disease) where dangerous respiratory depression is possible following lymphography. Therapeutic lung irradiation by paralysing lung capillaries, reduces the filtering ability of the lungs with a possible consequence of systemic embolisation; recent chest irradiation is therefore also a contraindication to lymphography.

Arteriography, the injection of contrast into major arteries, is not often required in malignant disease, though it may be important in localising tumours by demonstrating pathological circulations and stretching or displacement of normal vessels. It may be of value particularly in renal or adrenal lesions, in intracranial tumours and in certain bone tumours.

Mammography, the radiological examination of the breast tissues, is important in the demonstration and differential diagnosis of breast lumps and perhaps also in the screening of asymptomatic women. It is sometimes used in conjunction with *thermography* which makes use of infrared radiation emitted from the body; the thermographic image picked up by a heat sensitive scanner can be displayed visually as a thermogram on a cathode ray tube. Tumours near the skin surface (e.g. breast tumours) increase the skin temperature over the lesion compared with surrounding area—this shows as a hot spot on the thermogram.

Soft tissue radiography may be useful in identifying tumours, particularly sarcomas, which are interrupting or displacing normal tissue planes or eroding adjacent bony structures. It is also of considerable value, particularly when combined with tomography, in demonstrating tumours of the naso and laryngopharynx.

Ultrasonography, the use of high frequency (>50 kHz) sound waves in the diagnosis and management of tumours, is now assuming considerable importance as a non-invasive investigation. Ultrasound penetrates and interacts with tissues, and reflection of the incident ultrasound beam at interfaces between tissues of different density produces echos which can be translated into images on an oscilloscope; the images can be photographed and, in expert hands, are interpreted to give useful clinical information. Its major clinical role in oncology is in the assessment of the source and size of abdominal tumours. Lesions of the liver, spleen, kidney, abdominal lymph nodes and occasionally pancreas can be visualised.

Computerised axial tomography (CAT or CT scanning) is a non-invasive imaging technique in which a computer is used to reconstruct a two dimensional image from beams of X-rays directed through tissues of differing densities and hence different absorption coefficients. The use of transmission computerised tomography (first devised by EMI) is of established value in the diagnosis of lesions of the brain, but it has also been applied to the whole body with equally excellent results. Despite the major expenses in their installation, running and maintenance, CT scanners are becoming an established part of cancer investigation services.

Nuclear magnetic resonance (NMR), or magnetic resonance imaging (MRI), has recently undergone great advances in development, and has become a very valuable diagnostic tool. NMR imaging is based upon the fact that atomic nuclei with an odd number of protons and neutrons have intrinsic magnetism which endows them with the properties of bar magnets. When such nuclei are placed in a strong external magnetic field they become aligned with the lines of force. It is postulated that a little over half of the nuclei are disposed in one direction and a little under half in the opposite direction, so that there is a resultant net magnetic moment. An oscillating magnetic field applied in a plane at right angles to that of the first magnetic field will result in a change in the direction of alignment of the nuclei (rotation). Removal of this oscillating field will allow the nuclei to return to their former positions, and pulses of energy are released. These signals can be measured and can be characterised for the elemental nature of the nuclei concerned.

In medical NMR imaging, the amplitude of the signals recorded is proportional to the number of nuclei (protons) present. The signals can be recorded and displayed as an image of the tissues from which they have arisen. Transverse and longitudinal sections can be visualised, and enhancing techniques similar to those for CT scanning may be used.

The greater detail of tissue characterisation offers advantages over CT scanning, and the technique is being developed rapidly, with resultant increased excellence of the images obtained. The technique has the great advantage that no external irradiation is involved, and that to date no detrimental effects have been recorded.

Radioisotope scanning

Over the past 20 years, the use of radioisotopes in the investigation of malignant disease has made remarkable progress. The development of isotope generator systems, which continuously produce short-lived isotopes which can be kept in readiness in radioisotope departments, has greatly facilitated these investigations.

An isotope with a short half-life can be given in relatively high initial doses so that scanning shortly thereafter will yield a clearly defined scan print-out, without delivering an unacceptably high total radiation dose to the patient.

Developments in scanning equipment also have been marked. The earlier rectilinear scanners, as the name implies, scan backwards and forwards across the area, moving upwards or downwards a short distance between each sweep. They are slow in operation and require patients to lie stationary for relatively long periods. The newer gamma cameras record radiation picked up from the whole area of coverage simultaneously, and therefore are much quicker in use. Also, they can be used with the patient upright as well as horizontal.

The data obtained can be presented in two main forms. The signals from the scanner can be used to produce dots of blackening on photographic film, the density of the spots being proportional to the strength of the signal and hence to the amount of radiation received from the area monitored. The strength of the signal can also be used to determine the colour of a dot produced on a sheet of paper by a key registering on a multi-colour typewriter ribbon, or the colour of a small area on a multicolour cathode ray screen. If the latter technique is used, permanent records can be obtained by photographing the screen on colour film.

The isotopes used in imaging procedures must emit gamma radiation; alpha and beta rays have very short ranges in the tissues and measurements outside the body are seldom possible. The chemical form of the isotope must be such that the agent will be concentrated in or around the area to be scanned. In a few instances the agent is taken up preferentially by the tumour tissue, for example gallium; in most it is taken up solely or in greater amounts by the tissues around the tumour. Obviously, the chemical form of the isotope must be non-toxic, and must not produce any significant alteration in the normal tissue or organ physiology.

Radioiodine was the first isotope used extensively in the investigation of malignant disease, being applied to the study of thyroid function locally in the gland itself, and also generally, in an attempt to locate metastases from functioning thyroid carcinomas. Since then, many more isotopes have been added to the armamentarium of the radioisotope service. Table 2.1 lists the more commonly used isotopes, and indicates their half-lives and main applications.

Thyroid scanning. Iodine is an essential constituent of the thyroid hormone thyroxine, and most of the iodine absorbed from the gut gets to the gland. If radioiodine is available this will be taken up, and its amount and distribution in the thyroid tissue can be measured and depicted graphically. The rate of uptake and the rate of clearance of the isotope by the gland is of value as an assessment of thyroid function.

Table 2.1. Radioisotopes: half-lives and applications.

Isotope	Half-life	Main application
Iodine-131	8.06 days	Scanning of the thyroid and thyroid tumours
Iodine-132	2.29 hours	Assessment of thyroid function
Iodine-125	60.0 days	Thyroid hormone assays
Technetium-99m	6.02 hours	Bone, liver, lung and thyroid scanning
Gallium-67	78.26 hours	Tumour scanning (e.g. lymphoma, bronchus and seminoma)
Indium-113m	99.5 min	Brain and liver scanning
Selenium-75	118.5 days	Pancreatic and parathyroid scanning
Xenon-133	5.25 days	Ventilation lung scanning
Iodinated (I-131) human albumin	—	Perfusion lung scanning
Chromium-51	27.7 days	Red blood cell studies (e.g. polycythaemia)

In the investigation of malignant disease of the thyroid the distribution of isotope is important. Absence of uptake is an area (a so-called cold area) indicates non-functioning tissue which may be due to the presence of a carcinoma, cyst, non-functioning adenoma or an area of thyroiditis. Some well-differentiated tumours are able to take up iodine, but in much smaller amounts than the normal tissue. Nevertheless, if the competition of normal tissue is removed as by an ablation dose of radioiodine or by surgical total thyroidectomy, the relative uptake in tumour tissue will be increased, so that foci of tumour locally in the neck or in distant metastases may be demonstrable by scanning techniques.

An alternative isotope to radioiodine for scanning purposes is technetium-99m which is administered intravenously as pertechnetate.

Liver and spleen scanning. Radioisotopic scanning of the liver and spleen has become a very useful and common investigation in the management of malignant disease. It is simple and non-invasive, and with current equipment can demonstrate lesions as small as 1 cm in diameter.

Technetium-99m is the commonly used isotope. It is taken up by the lymphoreticular elements in the liver and spleen parenchyma following intravenous injection in the form of a colloid. Normally, these elements are evenly distributed and uptake is even. The presence of abnormal tissue, such as metastases or foci of lymphoma, shows as areas of reduced uptake.

Bone scanning. Scanning of localised areas or of the whole skeleton has provided a simple, easy and non-invasive technique for the detection of primary bone tumours or of metastases. For the detection and assessment of primary tumours, radiology remains supreme; for metastases, demonstration may be possible at a stage when no definite radiological changes are evident, and indeed before symptoms have developed. Radioisotope skeletal scanning is becoming of increasing value in the preliminary assessment of many tumours which have a tendency to metastasise early, the classical example being breast carcinoma.

The isotopes used are incorporated in the normal bone especially in areas of increased mineral turnover, as in bone adjacent to destructive lesions (metastases or primary tumour). Phosphate compounds labelled with technetium-99m are the most useful.

Brain scanning. As a simple non-invasive investigation brain scanning has proved to be a most useful addition to arteriography and ventriculography in the assessment of primary and secondary intracranial tumours. Again, technetium-99m is the isotope of choice. The scans differ from those obtained from most other organs in that the isotope escapes from the blood vessels in the tumour area thereby increasing the concentration in the tumour as compared with the normal brain tissue.

As a preliminary to technetium-99m scanning of the brain, a single oral dose of potassium chlorate is given to block uptake by the choroid plexuses and thereby limit the background radiation from them.

The clarity of demonstration of intracranial tumours depends mainly upon their vascularity. Poorly differentiated astrocytomas usually show up well; so also do meningiomas. The clarity of metastases varies; those with a good blood supply or those producing marked local oedema show well.

Lung scanning. Radioactive xenon-133 gas has been used to study the ventilatory efficiency of the lungs, and radioiodine-131 incorporated in minute particles of human albumin has been used to assess the blood flow through the lungs. These techniques have proved of some value, but are not routinely applied in oncology.

Isotopes taken up by tumours. Gallium-67 incorporated in plasma proteins is concentrated in tumour tissue, particularly lymphomas, and carcinomas of the bronchus and seminomas, and this isotope can be of value in the staging of tumours in these groups.

The amino acid analogue selenomethionine has been labelled with selenium-75 (half-life 118.5 days) and used to distinguish between benign and malignant space-occupying lesions in the liver, being selectively taken up by malignant lesions.

Chapter 3
Radiotherapy—
Principles and Practice

The origins of radiotherapy date back to the 1890s, when Becquerel discovered natural radioactivity, and Roentgen discovered X-rays. Following Becquerel's discovery the Curies' extracted a radiation-emitting element from pitchblende—radium.

It soon became evident that these radiations have a damaging effect on tissues, and that in some situations the damaging effect is greater for malignant tissues than for normal tissues. Before the turn of the century, the first malignant tumour had been treated successfully by irradiation—a basal cell carcinoma of the skin.

Since the momentous work of the Curies', many more radioactive elements have been discovered or produced artificially. Some have proved of immense value as sources of radiation for treatment purposes, and many have valuable applications as diagnostic tools.

Sources of X-rays and gamma-rays

X-rays are produced in electrical machines; the gamma-rays from radioactive elements emanate from the nuclei of the atoms of the elements. A wide range of energies of X-rays can be produced; the energy of naturally occurring radiation shows marked differences from one source to another. For practical purposes, however, there is no difference in the properties or effects between X-rays and gamma-rays of equivalent energies.

The radiation identified by Becquerel was of electromagnetic type (gamma-radiation). The nuclei of radioactive elements may also emit particulate radiation, consisting of particles composed of two protons and two neutrons (helium nuclei) called alpha-rays, and electrons called beta-rays. The beta-radiation from certain elements has a place, albeit limited, in the treatment of malignant disease; alpha-rays are of little if any value in this respect.

In addition to the particulate radiation from radioactive elements, it has become possible to accelerate subatomic particles in electrical machines, and to use these particles as defined beams for treatment purposes. The first such beams were of electrons, equivalent to high-energy beta-rays. More recently, it has become possible to generate beams of neutrons and of protons, and now beams of other particles are being investigated.

The unit of absorbed radiation dose

The unit by which the dose of radiation absorbed in tissue was quoted was the rad, which was defined as 100 ergs per gram of tissue at the point in question. With the introduction of the SI system of units, the basic unit became the gray (Gy); 1 centigray (cGy) is equilivent to 1 rad.

Modes of application of radiation therapy

The sources of the various radiations available have determined their chief modes of application. Beams of X-rays, and of gamma-rays from small high-activity sources, can be directed from without at tissue volumes in the body. Smaller radioactive sources, suitably mounted, can be applied to accessible body cavities, the best example of this technique being that of intracavitary treatment to a carcinoma of the uterine cervix. Radioactive elements as colloidal suspensions, or as soluble compounds in solution, have limited applications in closed body cavities such as the pleura and peritoneum, or by direct injection into the tissues.

Forms of radiation available

The forms of radiation currently available to the radiotherapist, and well established in practice, are shown in Table 3.1.

Table 3.1. Radiations used in the treatment of cancer.

X-RAYS

Grenz rays (10–15 kV energy)
Superficial X-rays (80–140 kV)
Deep X-rays (200–300 kV energy, sometimes termed orthovoltage X-rays)
Supervoltage or megavoltage X-rays (2–20 MV and above, but usually in the range of 4–8 MV)

RADIOISOTOPES

Alpha-rays (of little value)
Beta-rays (more penetrating, and of value for superficial areas)
Gamma-rays
(a) Small sealed sources
(b) High-activity sources, for external beam treatment (so-called teletherapy sources)

PARTICULATE BEAMS OF HIGH ENERGY

Electrons
Neutrons
Protons

Production of X-rays

X-rays are generated when electrons which have been accelerated across an evacuated tube between a heated filament (cathode) and a metal target (anode), interact with the electrons of the atoms in the target. The energy of this X-radiation is directly related to the energy of the incident electrons, which in turn is directly related to the electrical potential difference applied between the anode and cathode. For general radiotherapy the energy range is 10 kV to 8 MV.

Mode of action of X-rays and gamma-rays

When an X-ray or gamma-ray beam passes through tissue, ionisation is produced; this causes physiochemical changes in the cells of the tissue, resulting in damage to the intracellular mechanisms. Depending upon the site and the degree of the damage, recovery of function may or may not ensue; that is, the cells of the tissue may survive or may die. The energy absorbed from a beam by this ionisation process gradually reduces its residual energy, so that the dose delivered decreases with increasing depth of penetration.

Dose distribution in the tissues

For radiation generated at energies up to about 1 MV, the most intense ionisation is in the superficial tissues; the maximum dose is on the surface. At energies above 1 MV, the most intense ionisation is deep to the surface, with rapid build-up to a peak in the superficial layers and more gradual fall-off thereafter, the ionisation on the surface being relatively low. For 4 MV X-rays, the so-called build-up zone is about 1 cm, for 8 MV X-rays it is about 1.75 cm, and for cobalt-60 radiation it is about 0.5 cm.

Beyond the zone of maximum dose, the energy of an X-ray or gamma-ray beam is attenuated in an exponential manner, and the gradient of this absorption depends upon the energy of the incident beam. For low-energy X-ray beams in the range 10–140 kV, most of the energy is absorbed in the superficial layers of tissue, so that only very superficial volumes are treated adequately. At 10–15 kV energies the dose delivered even to the subcutaneous tissues by a beam applied directly to the skin surface is very low, and these energies of radiation have no place in the treatment of malignant conditions.

In the range 60–140 kV, the depth of adequate doseage is sufficient to treat superficial skin malignancies (basal and squamous cell carcinomas of limited infiltration).

X-rays generated in the energy range of 200–300 kV (orthovoltage) were the standard tool of the radiotherapist. Depth doses were adequate for the treatment of many malignancies, although to achieve a satisfactory total dose to a deeply situated tumour volume (e.g. carcinoma of the bladder or of the oesophagus) a relatively large number of convergent beams was necessary. The advent of supervoltage X-rays made it much easier to achieve an adequate total dose from three or four incident beams.

Teletherapy gamma-ray sources

The radiation from gamma-ray beam units is comparable with that from supervoltage X-ray machines. The two isotopes in general use are cobalt-60 and caesium-137. These emit radiation equivalent to about 3 MV and 600 kV X-rays respectively. One major practical difference between the X-ray and the gamma-ray units is that the radioisotopes gradually become less active, having specific half-lives for this activity. The half-life for cobalt-60 is 5.3 years; that for caesium-137 is 30.0 years.

Regular corrections for activity, and therefore for radiation output have to be made, and the sources have to be replaced when the output falls to levels at which treatment exposure times become unacceptably long. The output from X-ray machines remains fairly constant at all times.

Techniques of radiation beam therapy

Beams of X-rays or gamma-rays may be applied as a single direct beam, as an opposed pair of beams either tangentially to, or directly through, the tissues to be irradiated, or as multiple beams all convergent upon the volume to be irradiated.

For example, an accessible superficial area can be covered by a single direct beam (or field), and the energy can be relatively low, for example 100 kV, as for an early carcinoma of the skin. Higher energy beams, for example 4 MV X-rays or cobalt-60 gamma rays can be used for deeper areas.

In situations requiring irradiation of larger volumes of tissue, a parallel opposed pair of beams can be used. By this arrangement, the falling dose with increasing depth of penetration from one beam is countered by the falling dose from the opposite beam. Depending upon the energy of the beams, and upon the thickness of the tissue section the whole block may be fairly uniformly treated, for example using supervoltage X-rays and large fields.

Accurate application of beams

When a limited deeply situated volume is to be treated, for example a carcinoma of the middle third of the oesophagus, or a carcinoma of the bladder, multiple beams of radiation all directed at the required high-dose volume are needed. This requires precise application of beams.

Surface reference points can be marked on the skin surface if the patient can be positioned easily and comfortably so that immobility can be ensured, and if the skin is not lax and therefore not easily displaced. Otherwise, some form of mould or shell to fit the region accurately is necessary; usually this is made from cellulose acetate or similar material sheet.

Rotation therapy

Treatment machines which can be rotated about an horizontal axis through the centre of the treatment volume, have made it possible to use continuous rotation with the beam's central axis always passing through the centre of the volume, thus spreading the radiation dose to the skin surface over a band of skin around the body section instead of concentrating it over a few fixed areas of skin. With high-energy beams, the high-dose tissue volume can be fairly accurately confined, and if the tumour is near the centre of a body section, the dose distribution is also fairly homogenous. This technique has a limited application in radiation therapy.

Treatment simulators

Radiographs are of great value in verifying the extent and position of areas covered by radiation fields. A patient can be set up in each treatment position and the radiation from the therapy machine used to obtain the radiographs. However, all but the lowest energies used in the treatment of malignant disease produce poor quality films. Also, time which would be available for treatment exposures is used for the verifications. Therefore, units have been developed with the facility of reproducing treatment setups and using a diagnostic X-ray tube as the source of the radiation. Good quality films can be obtained, and valuable treatment time is not lost.

Treatment verification is still an important function of treatment simulators, but their main use now is the accurate localisation of the volume to be irradiated, that is, in the planning procedures, with verification of the field positions as the final part of the simulation.

CT scanning has proved of immense value in visualising the limits of tumour volumes, and not infrequently indicates wider limits than those assessed from other investigations. Furthermore, facilities are now available for superimposing, on the images of a CT scan picture, the positions of radiation beams and the resulting dose distribution. This may lead to greater accuracy and homogeneity of the high-dose distribution in the tissues.

Beta-ray therapy

The term beta-ray therapy is applied to the use of relatively low-energy electrons emitted by radioactive isotopes. The energies are such that the range of the electrons in the tissues is very limited, being of the order of 3–5 mm. Beta-ray sources can therefore be used as surface applicators or plaques to treat very superficial lesions such as port-wine stain type haemangiomas (if in fact radiation therapy is indicated), or as surface contact solutions or colloidal suspensions in body cavities such as the pleural and peritoneal spaces to treat effusions due to thin layers of tumour on these surfaces. In the latter applications they are termed 'unsealed sources'. The limited depth of penetration confines their use to such superficial lesions; they are of no value in the treatment of malignant skin tumours or of bulkier tumour deposits on serous surfaces.

The isotopes used for surface applicators include strontium-90 and phosphorus-32. Isotopes used for intracavitary instillation include yttrium-90 (in solution as its chloride salt) and gold-198 (as colloidal suspension of elemental gold).

The systemic administration of phosphorus-32 for polycythaemia vera falls within the category of unsealed source therapy; so also does the use of iodine-131 in the management of thyrotoxicosis and thyroid malignancy.

Small sealed sources

Small sealed gamma-ray sources have been used since the earliest days of radiotherapy. The commonest types are needles and tubes, initially containing radium-226 as its chloride or sulphate salt in dry powder form, but more recently also available containing caesium-137. Radium emits alpha, beta and gamma-rays; caesium-137 emits beta and gamma-rays only.

Needles are thin hollow metal tubes, with a blunt point at one end and an eyelet at the other end, containing one or more thin-walled metal capsules in which the radioactive powder is packed. The needle body is made of a platinum-iridium alloy and the capsules are made of gold. The eyelet carries a silk thread which is used in handling the needle at a distance and in extracting it from the tissues when the treatment time has expired, and the colour of the silk can be coded to indicate the activity of the needle.

Capsules are used to ensure uniform distribution of the radioactive powder along the length of the needle by limiting the amount of 'settling' of the powder which might occur from prolonged storage when not in use, and also to ease the loading of needles of different lengths during manufacture.

For implantation (interstitial) treatments, use is made of the gamma-radiation only. Any alpha or beta-radiation would produce a very high local dose close to the needle without contributing to the irradiation of a wider tumour area. The alpha-radiation is easily absorbed in the thin gold wall of the inner capsule, and the beta-radiation is absorbed in the wall of the body of the needle. The platinum-iridium alloy also has the advantage that it is non-toxic to the tissues, and that it has a very high melting point; the latter is an advantage especially if a needle accidentally gets into an incinerator with soiled dressings, as might occasionally occur.

The half-life of radium is approximately 1600 years; therefore, any correction for decay of activity is insignificant over the useful lifetime of the needle or tube containing it. The half-life of caesium-137 is 30.0 years, and regular corrections for decay are essential.

Radiocaesium-137 is the isotope now commonly used for intracavitary treatment of carcinoma of the uterine cervix and body, and it is usual practice to correct the activity figures every 6 months.

Tubes are similar in structure to needles, but are shorter and broader. They do not need a point at the end, but may have an eyelet at one end to take a silk thread for handling and identification purposes. Usually they are mounted in applicators for intracavitary treatments.

For permanent implantation small radioactive gold-198 pellets (gold grains) are available. They have a half-life of 2.7 days. They emit beta and gamma-radiation, and are ensheathed in platinum which absorbs the beta-rays. The short half-life means that most of the activity decays in the first week, and is virtually zero after 1 month. They are chemically inert in the tissues.

The radioisotope iridium-192 is a metal and is available as wire which can be cut into any required length for introduction into the tissues in much the same way as radium needles. It has a half-life of 74 days, and emits beta and gamma-radiation; the beta-radiation is absorbed in a sheath of platinum, as with gold grains.

Application of small sealed sources

Radioactive needles can be used to treat superficial tumours in accessible sites, the classical example being that of a localised and superficial carcinoma on the lateral border of the tongue. The needles have to be left *in situ* for the calculated period of time to deliver the required dose; this is usually 6 or 7 days.

Intracavitary radiocaesium therapy to carcinomas of the uterine cervix and body is considered in Chapter 10.

An example of a gold grain implant is the treatment of a localised and superficial well-differentiated transitional cell carcinoma of the urinary bladder, beyond the scope of eradication by diathermy and not requiring cystectomy. Once implanted at open operation the radiation sources do not have to be removed at a second operation.

Iridium-192 wire has been used, for example, to treat superficial areas on the body surface, such as a plaque of recurrent tumour on the chest wall after mastectomy for breast carcinoma, and has been implanted into the lateral border of the tongue to treat a carcinoma in this site, as an alternative to radium or radiocaesium needles.

Electron beam therapy

The term electron therapy is usually applied to the use of defined beams of high-energy electrons produced in electrical machines, and applied in much the same way as single beams of X-rays or gamma-rays. However, the range of electrons in the tissues is finite and is related to the energy of the incident beam.

The dose delivered in the tissues is constant within ± 10% to a depth of about two-thirds of the maximum electron range. Therefore, virtually homogenous doses can be delivered to defined blocks of tissue to a depth determined by the energy of the beam, with little radiation dose beyond the high-dose volume.

Electron beams are of value in the treatment of some tumours in the head and neck region, for example. The useful range of energies is about 10–35 MeV; 20 MeV electrons have a treatment range of 5 cm.

Neutron beam therapy

In larger tumour masses the central areas may be necrotic because of absence of blood vessels, and cells in these areas die. Towards the periphery of tumours blood supply is usually good. In a zone between these two the degree of oxygenation may be just adequate to allow the cells to survive, but low enough to reduce their sensitivity to X- or gamma-radiation by a factor of three. This concept has been used to explain the limited response of larger tumour masses, and the relatively high incidence of residual or recurrent tumour in them after radiation therapy. These effects will be augmented if the patient is anaemic.

However, the damaging effects of high-energy neutrons, referred to as fast neutrons, are much less influenced by the degree of oxygenation of the tissues, and the difference between good oxygenation and anoxia is a factor of only 1.6 or so. Interest in their use in the treatment of tumours has increased rapidly over the past 20 years. The sensitivity of fully oxygenated normal cells to damage by fast neutrons is not altered.

This low dependence on oxygenation of cellular damage by neutrons is related to the mode of interaction with the atoms of the cell constituents. Whereas X-radiation and gamma-radiation interact with the electron layers of atoms, with ejection of electrons which produce sparse ionisations and which require the presence of oxygen for full effect, neutrons interact with atomic nuclei with ejection of protons and other heavy particles which produce much denser ionisations which are much less affected by the presence or absence of oxygen.

Another factor is the degree of recovery from cellular damage which occurs between each exposure of a treatment course. The less dense ionisations of X-irradiation and gamma-irradiation produce less severe damage at each exposure and more recovery occurs; recovery from the denser ionisations and more severe damage of neutron irradiation is less marked.

To be of use in the treatment of tumours neutron beams must be sufficiently penetrating and sufficiently dense to deliver the required dose in an acceptably short treatment time. At the present time such beams are generated in massive machines called cyclotrons, positive ions being accelerated and directed at a target of a low atomic number element (e.g. beryllium), resulting in the expulsion of neutrons. An alternative method is the interaction between accelerated deuterons and a tritium target. Machines using the latter principle are smaller, simpler and cheaper than cyclotrons, and are much more versatile as regards the ease of setting up patients for treatment. However, the tube in which the interactions occur has a short life, and the neutron beam produced is less intense than that from a cyclotron.

With the development of acceptable treatment schedules it has become apparent that the responses to neutron therapy can be superior to those with photon (X-ray or gamma-ray) therapy, especially in tissues which have been regarded as resistant to the latter form of treatment. Good responses in gastric adenocarcinoma and soft-tissue sarcomas have been reported. Responses in other relatively radioresistant tumours have been disappointing, for example in high-grade astrocytomas, in chondrosarcomas and in colorectal adenocarcinomas.

To date, experience with fast neutron therapy has been confined to the palliative treatment of advanced tumours, and its place as a possible alternative to X-ray and gamma-ray therapy in the radical treatment of earlier tumours has yet to be determined.

Proton beam therapy

Beams of high-energy protons have a limited place in radiotherapy. Protons have the same mass as neutrons, but whereas neutrons are electrically neutral protons carry unit positive charge. Like other accelerated particles protons have a finite maximum range in the tissues, this being dependent upon the incident energy. Protons of 100 MeV energy have an average tissue range of about 10 cm. However, the energy distribution along the track of a proton in the tissues is different; the energy imparted is relatively low for most of the track, but as the particle slows down the energy imparted rises rapidly. Thus, the so-called 'linear energy transfer' is highly concentrated at the end of the particle's path. This localised high intensity of ionisation can be made to coincide with a tumour volume to be treated, provided this is small, by selecting an appropriate incident energy, and has been used, for example, in the treatment of pituitary tumours. Proton beams can be generated in cyclotrons; very high energies are required, and the beams are narrow.

Hyperbaric oxygen and radiotherapy

The presence of hypoxic or anoxic cells in larger tumour masses, and the effect of oxygen deficiency on the radiosensitivity of these cells has been discussed (see p. 40). The amount of oxygen available to such cells may be increased by increasing the oxygenation of their blood supply. Under normal conditions, the haemoglobin is almost saturated with oxygen, and the amount in the blood can be increased only by increasing the amount of oxygen in simple solution in the plasma. Breathing pure oxygen at atmospheric pressure increases the arterial oxygen content very little, but a significant rise can be achieved at a pressure of 3 atm (304 kPa). In practice, this is the maximum pressure tolerated by an unanaesthetised person.

Nevertheless, a conscious patient can be enclosed in a pressure vessel, filled with pure oxygen, and the pressure raised to three times that of the atmosphere. This technique requires repeated pressurisations, and the technical difficulties, quite apart from the psychological aspects, are great. The number of treatment exposures has to be reduced below the usual schedule of five times each week, and treatment techniques must be simplified.

Improved results have been reported from some randomised trials of hyperbaric oxygen therapy, but not from others, and the technique is not firmly established in general radiotherapy practice.

Radiosensitisers

About 13 years ago, first reports were published of investigations into the radiosensitising effects of so-called electron-affinic agents on hypoxic cells. These agents appear to mimic the radiobiological action of oxygen without being metabolised. They can diffuse into avascular areas.

They must be non-toxic, or only mildly so. They must be simple to administer, preferably by mouth, and be well absorbed.

Currently, benznidazole is being investigated. It has been shown to have a sensitising or potentiating effect for cytotoxic chemotherapy agents, as well as for radiation, *in vivo*.

After-loading techniques

The handling of sealed sources of radiation for interstitial or intracavitary therapy exposes the operator and other staff in close proximity to a relatively small but finite radiation dose. The amount of this dose will depend upon the activity of the sources, the distances of the sources from the individuals and the time of the exposure. The last factor will depend upon the dexterity of the operator and the complexity of the manoeuvres involved. With practice the time taken for procedures will be reduced.

Nevertheless, any reasonably obtained reduction in the exposure of staff to irradiation is to be commended and with this aim after-loading techniques have been developed. These require the insertion of applicator holders into the area to be treated, for example, vagina, uterine cavity, side of tongue, or tissues of the chest wall. Radio-opaque dummy sources are then inserted, and the positions checked radiologically, and modified if necessary, after which the dummy sources are replaced by active ones.

In some techniques the insertion of the radioactive sources is done manually; in others it is done mechanically by remote control, as in the Cathetron and Selectron systems. For the latter techniques, highly active sources can be used so that insertion times are short, but this requires a specially protected room for the treatment.

Fractionation in radiotherapy

Just as normal cells of different tissues are not all equally sensitive to the damaging effects of ionising radiation, so the cells of different tumours differ in their sensitivity to such damage. Furthermore, the sensitivity of any particular tumour cell type varies with the phase of the cell cycle at which it is irradiated. Cells are most sensitive immediately before mitosis.

In a mixed population of cells all will not be at the same stage of the cycle at the same time. If, however, repeated radiation exposures are given, more cells will be irradiated at the most sensitive phase and more cells will be killed.

The use of multiple exposures in radiotherapy is termed fractionation, and is applied to the treatment of most malignant conditions. Sometimes, a single exposure of superficial X-rays is used for a small superficial basal or squamous cell carcinoma of the skin, but the cosmetic results are inferior to those from fractionated treatment, and the risks of late tissue breakdown are greater.

Fractionated treatments may range in number from 4 or 5 to 25 or more, depending on the type of malignancy and the volume of tissue concerned, and on the total dose to be delivered. Usually, treatment exposures are given daily from Monday to Friday each week. Sometimes, thrice weekly treatments are used—Monday, Wednesday and Friday—and occasionally once weekly schedules are used.

Radiosensitivity of tumours

The differing degrees of sensitivity to radiation damage shown by the cells of different tumours makes it possible to divide them broadly into three groups, termed 'radiosensitive', 'limited sensitivity' and 'radioresistant'. It must be stressed, however, that these terms are not absolute, there being some variation within each group, and some degree of overlap between the groups. Nevertheless, the subdivisions in Table 3.2 are useful.

Table 3.2. Examples of the radiosensitivity of tumours.

RADIOSENSITIVE TUMOURS

Malignant lymphomas
Seminoma of the testis
Medulloblastoma, neuroblastoma, Wilms' tumour (nephroblastoma)

TUMOURS OF LIMITED SENSITIVITY

Squamous cell and basal cell carcinomas of the skin
Carcinomas of the mouth, including tongue and lip
Carcinomas of the accessory nasal sinuses
Carcinoma of the bladder
Carcinoma of the larynx

RADIORESISTANT TUMOURS

Osteosarcoma
Fibrosarcoma, liposarcoma and the myosarcomas
Malignant melanoma
Large bowel adenocarcinomas
Gliomas

Radiosensitive tumours

In general, the radiosensitive tumours respond well to radiotherapy, which may be effective alone, or may require the addition of cytotoxic chemotherapy as in the more advanced stages of Hodgkin's disease and Wilms' tumour. Indeed, for some malignancies which have a tendency to disseminate early, cytotoxic therapy has the major role in the initial definitive treatment regimens with greatly improved results. For example, the addition of cytotoxic therapy to surgical excision and radiotherapy for Wilms' tumour has resulted in a rise in the chance of normal life-expectancy from about 30% to about 90% overall. The comparable figures for advanced Hodgkin's disease are from about 5% to about 45% overall.

Tumours of limited sensitivity

The term 'tumours of limited sensitivity' is a useful one. The total dose of radiation tolerated by normal tissues decreases as the volume irradiated increases. The tumours in this group are sufficiently sensitive to be curable in many cases if the volume to be irradiated is small and tolerance high, but not so if the volume is larger and tolerance correspondingly lower. An example is that of an early localised carcinoma in the faucial region of the mouth, with a curability of about 75%, as compared with a more advanced local lesion with inoperable lymph node deposits in the neck, which is curable in only a few instances.

Radioresistant tumours

Tumours in the radioresistant group show some slight variations in their level of response to irradiation, but in general all would require doses in excess of local tissue tolerances to produce any significant response. Therefore they cannot be eradicated by this form of treatment; surgical excision, if possible, offers the only chance of cure. Nevertheless, some show partial responses to irradiation, and this form of treatment can offer useful palliation of otherwise untreatable malignancies in carefully selected cases. The availability of cytotoxic therapy has improved the prospects in some malignancies in this group using combined treatment regimens.

Effects on normal tissues: radiation reactions

The damaging effects of radiation are induced in normal as well as abnormal tissues. Under favourable circumstances these effects can be lethal to tumour cells and sub-lethal to normal cells, so that the tumour cells are killed whereas the normal cells can recover. However, all normal tissues have a level of damage beyond which recovery does not occur; this is termed the 'tolerance dose'.

Many treatment situations require the use of doses approaching the tolerance doses of normal tissues in the treatment volume, so that inevitably there will be significant damage to them. This damage is evident clinically as the 'radiation reaction' in the skin and mucous membranes within high dose volumes. The reaction follows much the same course in both skin and mucosa, first being evident between 2 and 3 weeks from the start of treatment as erythema of the skin and injection of the mucosa. Over the next 2 weeks the intensity of the reaction gradually increases. In the skin this leads to scaling (dry desquamation) and a variable degree of pigmentation, and may progress to superficial desquamation with serous exudation (moist desquamation). In the mucosa it leads to an exudation with the formation of a fibrinous deposit (fibrinous reaction). In both situations, there is associated discomfort and soreness towards the height of the reaction; a mucosal reaction in the pharynx or oesophagus will be associated with dysphagia, in the rectum it will be associated with tenesmus and diarrhoea, and in the bladder it will be associated with frequency and dysuria.

Skin and mucosal reactions usually reach their height by the fifth week, and gradually subside thereafter over a period of a further 3 or 4 weeks.

Relatively low doses of radiation will produce epilation. Usually this becomes evident during the third week, and hair regrowth usually commences after 2 or 3 months. Higher doses may result in permanent epilation, and certainly this is to be expected from doses approaching tolerance of the skin.

After longer periods other changes become apparent. Skin which has received full-dose treatment becomes thinner and smoother, hair follicles and sweat glands become scanty, and telangiectases develop. Such skin is more liable to breakdown if damaged, even by sunlight or cold, and may be slow to heal—so-called late radiation necrosis. Late malignant change in heavily irradiated skin occurs occasionally. Mucous membranes in high-dose areas also become somewhat atrophic and their natural secretions reduced; again telangiectases may develop. In subcutaneous tissues fibrosis develops and may become well marked.

Other irradiated normal tissues also manifest radiation damage but the effects are usually not so clinically obvious. However, some are very easily damaged, for example the cornea and lens of the eye, the salivary glands, the lung parenchyma, the brain and spinal cord tissues, and the renal tissues. If any of these tissues are within a volume to be irradiated the total dose delivered must be reduced appropriately.

Healthy teeth do not show any evidence of direct radiation damage. Irradiation of the gums, however, results in some recession around the necks of the teeth which thus become exposed, and if salivary tissue is also within the high-dose volume the quality of the saliva changes and this predisposes to dental caries. If there are carious teeth in a volume to be treated it is beneficial to remove these before starting radiotherapy, unless the delay would be unacceptable.

The haemopoietic tissues of the body are also very susceptible to radiation damage. The irradiation of large volumes containing red bone marrow will result in falls in the peripheral blood leucocyte and platelet counts, and these falls may limit the total dose which can be delivered. Immunosuppression may be severe. Changes in the haemoglobin level are much less and are much slower to develop.

When large volumes are irradiated general effects are evident in the form of so-called radiation sickness. This is a syndrome of nausea, vomiting, and general lethargy. It is related to the actual volume of tissue treated, and also to the site treated—being more marked if the upper abdomen is within the field. Its severity is also related to the rate at which treatment is given.

Management of radiation reactions

Skin reactions

The management of skin reaction to radiation commences with the start of radiation treatment. The irradiated area should be kept dry and exposed to the air as much as possible. Local application is restricted to bland talcum powder (without added perfume or antiperspirant) unless moist desquamation develops, when a protective and mildly antiseptic application is permissible. For the latter, the time-honoured 0.5% aqueous gentian violet solution still has its advocates; others prefer 0.5% cetrimide cream. Moist desquamation in skin near the eye can be treated with a steroid-antibiotic eye ointment. Since skin which is reacting is delicate, clothing in contact with it should be soft and non-irritant.

Mucosal reactions

The management of mucosal reactions depends upon the site, but a high fluid intake is vital in all cases. In the mouth, frequent bland mouth washes (e.g. dilute sodium bicarbonate solution) are indicated from the start of radiotherapy; this helps to keep the mouth clean and free of food particles and exudate. Later, a mouth wash with mildly antiseptic effects is helpful. Not infrequently, mouth reactions are complicated by monilial infections, in which case an antifungal agent is required (e.g. nystatin). Pharyngeal reactions produce dysphagia and soothing mixtures (e.g. an antacid mixture containing a topical anaesthetic) are helpful when taken before meals. In the later stages, antibiotics can be of benefit, and oxytetracyline in particular is effective.

Bladder mucosal reactions

In the management of bladder mucosal reactions, a good fluid intake and hence good urinary output, is essential. The urine must be checked regularly for the presence of infection, which if detected must be appropriately treated.

Bowel reactions

Bowel reactions may lead to troublesome diarrhoea. Again, a good fluid intake is essential, together with an antidiarrhoeal preparation (e.g. kaolin and morphine mixture, or codeine phosphate) or an antispasmodic preparation (e.g. loperamide) given with due caution. Rectal mucosal reactions are aggravated by the presence of hard faeces, and a small dose of liquid paraffin by mouth each morning may prove very effective in softening and lubricating the lower bowel contents.

Radical or palliative treatment

In the treatment of malignant disease, it is important to determine in each individual case whether cure of the disease is possible or probable. If cure is likely, the inevitable side effects and local reactions to treatment are more than justifiable. On the other hand, if cure is unlikely, it is vital that treatment offers improvement in the symptoms present, without the addition or substitution of significant symptoms from the treatment itself, and the probable side effects and local reactions to treatment must be carefully weighed against the expected benefits. This applies equally well to all forms of cancer therapy.

Chapter 4
Cytotoxic Chemotherapy—
Principles and Practice

The great surgeon Bilroth first used chemotherapy, in the form of arsenic, in an attempt to cure his patients with lymphoma, but it was not until following World War I that the effects of mustard gas on bone marrow cells were reported and gratifying responses of lymphoid neoplasms to nitrogen mustard were seen.

Many chemically related compounds were then screened and tested, and later in the 1940s methotrexate and other antimetabolite drugs were discovered. Since then over half a million new chemicals have been tested but no more than three dozen are in present-day regular clinical use.

Nowadays any potentially cytotoxic drug is screened in animal systems for tumouricidal effects and for toxic effects. Clinical trials for a drug passing this stage are in three phases:

1 Clinical pharmacological studies in patients with advanced cancer.

2 Administration to groups of patients with specific tumours to identify responsiveness.

3 Administration to larger numbers of patients, with a range of responsive neoplasms, by differing schedules and routes of administration to establish its role in the treatment of a tumour.

After these studies sufficient clinical information will be available on the drug as a single agent; it can then be tried in combination regimens to ascertain its full effectiveness.

Pharmacology

As for all drugs the absorption, distribution, metabolism and excretion of chemotherapeutic agents must be considered. Absorption of oral drugs may be altered by the presence of cancer, by changes in the patient's dietary habits and by changes in bowel motility, as well as by other drugs being simultaneously ingested. Also in many cases cytotoxic drugs are degraded by enzymes in the stomach and small intestine or may be intensely irritant to the intestinal mucosa. The oral route is therefore the most unreliable, particularly since it also depends on patient compliance.

Once in the body, hepatic and tissue metabolism, distribution into body compartments and renal excretion must also be considered. Passage of drugs across the blood–brain barrier and their penetration into large tumours with hypoxic and necrotic centres may be important. The presence of pleural or peritoneal effusions will act as an extra compartment for the distribution of many agents.

For the attainment of effective levels of most cytotoxic drugs the intravenous (rapid injection or continuous infusion) route is best, though the intramuscular route may be suitable in some cases (e.g. with bleomycin and thiotepa). Palliative relief of pleural effusions and ascites can be obtained by intracavity instillation of drugs (e.g. nitrogen mustard, bleomycin, thiotepa).

Intrathecal therapy (with, for example, methotrexate in leukaemia) is necessary when good cerebrospinal fluid (CSF) levels of the drug are vital, but the number of drugs that can be given in this way is very limited.

Intra-arterial infusion was popular a few years ago but is now thought to be largely ineffective except in occasional cases. Topical and intralesional cytotoxics are also of occasional value.

Biochemical classifications of cytotoxic drugs

A list of the commonly used cytotoxic drugs with biochemical and kinetic classifications and usual routes of administration is given in Table 4.1. The sites of action of some of the agents are shown in Fig. 4.1.

Alkylating agents

The main chemical reaction in this group of drugs is the formation of a covalent bond between highly reactive alkyl groups of the drug and a nitrogen group of guanine. The cross-linking of the guanine groups of the DNA helix either prevents division of the helix at mitosis or results in imperfect division with malunion. Fragmentation or clumping of chromosomes, and hence cell death, may result. Enzymes concerned with DNA synthesis may also be alkylated thus preventing the formation of new DNA chains. Some drugs in this group are more effective because they have two or more alkyl radicals (bifunctional or polyfunctional agents).

Mustine (nitrogen mustard) was the first agent to be used clinically, but it is very toxic. It is given intravenously (i.v.) since it causes tissue necrosis on direct contact. The drug is extensively metabolised and rapidly tissue bound and it is excreted via the liver and the kidney; it has a short plasma half-life.

Table 4.1. Commonly used cytotoxic drugs (trade name in brackets).

Biochemical group and drug	Cycle or phase specificity	Route
ALKYLATING AGENTS		
Mustine hydrochloride		i.v., i.c.
Cyclophosphamide (Endoxana)		i.v., oral
Ifosfamide (Mitoxana)		i.v.
Chlorambucil (Leukeran)	Cycle	oral, i.v.
Melphalan (Alkeran)		oral
Busulphan (Myleran)		oral
Thiotepa		i.m., i.c.
Nitrosoureas		oral, i.v.
ANTIMETABOLITES		
Methotrexate	Phase	i.v., oral, i.m., i.t.
Pyrimidine analogues:		
Fluorouracil	Cycle	i.v., oral
Cytarabine (Cytosar)	Phase	i.v.
Purine analogues:		
Mercaptopurine (Puri-Nethol)	Phase	
Thioguanine (Lanvis)	Cycle	oral
Azathioprine (Imuran)	Cycle	
VINCA ALKALOIDS		
Vincristine (Oncovin)		
Vinblastine (Velbe)	Phase	i.v.
Vindesine (Eldisine)		
ANTIBIOTICS		
Actinomycin D	Cycle	i.v.
Daunorubicin (Daunomycin)	Cycle	i.v.
Doxorubicin (Adriamycin)	Cycle	i.v.
Epirubicin (Pharmarubicin)	Cycle	i.v.
Bleomycin	Phase	i.v., i.m.
Mitozantrone (Novantrone)	Cycle	i.v.
ENZYMES		
Asparaginase (Colospase)	Phase	i.v.
MISCELLANEOUS		
Procarbazine (Natulan)	Phase	oral
Hydroxyurea	Phase	oral, i.v.
Dacarbazine (DTIC)	Cycle	i.v.
Hexamethylmelamine	Cycle	oral
Razoxane	Phase	oral
Cisplatin (Neoplatin)	Cycle	i.v.
Etoposide (Vepesid)	Phase	oral, i.v.
Glucocorticoids	Phase	oral

i.v. intravenous; i.m. intramuscular; i.c. intracavity; i.t. intrathecal.

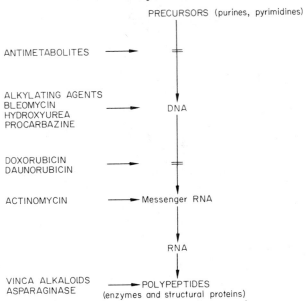

Fig. 4.1. Principal sites of biochemical action of cytotoxic drugs in common use.

Cyclophosphamide may be given i.v. or orally. Its cytotoxic action is via active hepatic metabolites. The plasma half-life is about 4 hours and it is excreted via both liver and kidneys.

Ifosfamide is related to cyclophosphamide; it is activated by liver microsomal enzymes and the metabolites excreted by the kidneys. Urothelial toxicity (also seen with higher doses of cyclophosphamide) is a problem which is reduced by administering *mesna*, which reacts specifically with the urotoxic metabolite acrolein in the urinary tract.

Chlorambucil is well absorbed after oral administration with a plasma half-life of less than half an hour. Its pharmacokinetics are mostly unknown.

Melphalan (phenylalanine mustard) is well absorbed orally, has a plasma half-life of 4 hours and is extensively metabolised in the tissues. It has proved particularly useful in myeloma treatment.

Busulphan, extensively used in chronic myeloid leukaemia, is well absorbed orally but has a very short plasma half-life (a few minutes) and is excreted in the urine.

Thiotepa is usually given by intramuscular (i.m.) injection because of its unpredictable gastrointestinal absorbtion. It has a half-life of about 3 hours, is extensively metabolised and is excreted mainly via the kidneys.

Nitrosoureas. *Carmustine*—BCNU   (1,3-bis-2-chlorethyl-1-nitrosourea); *lomustine*—CCNU; and the less commonly used *semustine* (methyl CCNU) are usually classified as alkylating agents. They are lipid soluble and cross the blood–brain barrier. Carmustine is given i.v.; lomustine is well absorbed orally. Bone marrow toxicity may be delayed for 3–4 weeks after treatment with these compounds and little is known of their pharmacokinetic properties.

Other less commonly used alkylating drugs include *treosulphan*, *estramustine* (a stable combination of mustine and oestrogen), *mitobronitol* and *mitolactol*.

Antimetabolites

These compounds closely resemble metabolites essential to the synthesis of nucleic acids and proteins. They are therefore incorporated into natural metabolic pathways and enzyme systems; the products however differ functionally from the intended natural products, resulting in either the inhibition of subsequent enzyme systems or in the formation of biologically inactive nuclear proteins; cell division is therefore prevented. Each antimetabolite acts at different sites in the nucleic acid synthesis pathways.

Methotrexate is a folic acid antagonist; it inactivates the enzyme dihydrofolate reductase which normally reduces dihydrofolate to tetrahydrofolate, the precursor of active metabolites. The latter compounds, essential coenzymes in the formation of purines and pyrimidines, are therefore depleted and precursor synthesis is halted. Methotrexate may be given orally, but to achieve high plasma levels (e.g. in pulse therapy) intravenous bolus or infusion is essential. The drug is not metabolised but is extensively protein and tissue bound. It is excreted mainly in the urine and also in the bile. Serious side effects can be reduced by folinic acid rescue (see p. 64).

Pyrimidine analogues. The two most important pyrimidine antimetabolites are *fluorouracil* and *cytarabine* (cytosine arabinoside). The former exerts its antimitotic activity by blocking the enzyme thymidilate synthetase in the DNA pathway and also by inhibiting incorporation of uracil into RNA. It is given i.v., or less reliably by mouth; it is extensively metabolised and excreted in the urine, with a half-life of about 30 minutes. Cytarabine probably acts on DNA polymerase, an enzyme vital to the final steps of DNA strand assembly. This drug is given i.v. and has a short plasma half-life. After being metabolised it is excreted by the kidneys.

Purine analogues. Of the purine analogues *mercaptopurine* is probably the most important. It acts by blocking adenine and guanine synthesis in the DNA pathway. Gastrointestinal absorption is good, metabolisation rapid and excretion via the urine. *Thioguanine* (sometimes used in leukaemia protocols) and *azathioprine* (an immunosuppressive compound used in transplant procedures and autoimmune disorders) are also well absorbed after oral administration.

Vinca alkaloids

Vincristine and vinblastine vary only slightly in their chemical structure, but have differences in their antimitotic activity and in adverse effects. They are derived from the periwinkle plant, *Vinca rosea*. The main site of action of the drugs is at the metaphase of mitosis, probably by toxicity to the microtubules of the mitotic spindle. Both drugs are given i.v. and have short plasma half-lives (less than 1 hour). After extensive metabolism excretion is mainly biliary. *Vindesine*, a new synthetic vinca alkaloid derived from vinblastine, acts in a similar way to vincristine and vinblastine and has toxic effects somewhere between these agents.

Antibiotics

Many antibiotics, mainly from the *Streptomyces* genus, have been found to inhibit tumour cell division. *Actinomycin D* forms irreversible complexes with DNA strands; the main effect is to block DNA-dependent RNA synthesis. The mechanism of action of *doxorubicin* and *daunorubicin* is probably similar to that of actinomycin D but the action of *bleomycin* is less clearly understood, though it is known to fragment DNA chains, thus interfering with DNA replication.

Antibiotic cytotoxic agents are usually given by i.v. injection since gastrointestinal absorption is unreliable. Bleomycin is an exception in that it may be given i.m. The plasma half-life of these drugs is generally short (less than half an hour) as they quickly disappear into the tissues. Actinomycin D, daunorubicin and doxorubicin are mainly excreted via the bile. Bleomycin is excreted in the urine.

Other antibiotics, less important clinically at the present time, are *mitomycin* and *mithramycin*. Mitomycin is a relatively toxic drug; it causes delayed marrow toxicity. Its clinical use is therefore limited. Mithramycin is not now used as a cytotoxic drug but has a place in the emergency treatment of malignant hypercalcaemia.

Newly introduced drugs include *epirubicin* which seems to be less cardiotoxic than the related doxorubicin, and *amsacrine* (which is similar in action and toxicity to doxorubicin). *Mitozantrone* is a synthetic anthracenedione structurally related to doxorubicin, which appears to act by intercalation with DNA.

Enzymes

L-asparaginase promised in theory to be an important antitumour agent. It acts by breaking down asparagine, an amino acid essential to all human cells, but not synthesised by tumour cells. In practice the drug proved disappointing. It has a role to play in acute leukaemia but is rather toxic, one problem being the hypersensitivity reactions to the drug.

Miscellaneous drugs

Procarbazine is a monoamine oxidase (MAO) inhibitor given orally which acts primarily on DNA, partly by causing fragmentation of strands and partly by an antimetabolic action. As with all MAO inhibitors drug interactions (e.g with anaesthetic agents, phenothiazines, alcohol) are not uncommon. It has a short plasma half-life and is excreted in the urine.

Hydroxyurea is a simple drug of short plasma half-life administered orally or i.v.; it interferes with ribonucleotide reductase and thus inhibits DNA synthesis.

Etoposide, an epipodophyllotoxin derived alkaloid, interferes with microtubule assembly thus inhibiting mitosis. It is mainly excreted in the urine. A similar agent *teniposide* is also currently being evaluated.

The mode of action and pharmacokinetics of *razoxane, hexamethylmelamine, dacarbazine* and *cisplatin* are incompletely understood, though the latter three drugs seem to have an alkylating action. Dacarbazine and cisplatin are given i.v. Razoxane and hexamethylmelamine are given orally but are used only infrequently. A new platinum derivative (*carboplatin*) appears to be better tolerated than the toxic cisplatin and is undergoing extensive clinical trials.

Glucocorticoids seem to have a definite antitumour effect, acting at an early stage of the cell cycle and interfering with DNA synthesis. Prednisolone (or prednisone) given orally is often used in combination chemotherapy, particularly of the leukaemias and lymphomas. Steroids are also specifically indicated for certain complications of malignancy (e.g. hypercalcaemia, cerebral oedema, haemolytic anaemia); their side effects are well known.

Kinetic classification

The body's cells can be divided into three compartments (stem cells, differentiating cells and dead cells). The stem cell compartment is the smallest and has the capacity for indefinite cell division. Differentiating cells have a limited capacity for division. Both differentiating and stem cells take part in the normal cell cycle, but it is usually the malignant stem cell population at which cancer chemotherapy is primarily aimed.

Experiments have shown that cytotoxic drugs may act at different phases of the cell cycle (phase specific) or alternatively may act throughout the cell cycle (cycle specific). Most drugs fall into the latter group (see Table 4.1). Some examples of the sites of action in the cell cycle of phase-specific drugs are illustrated in Fig. 4.2.

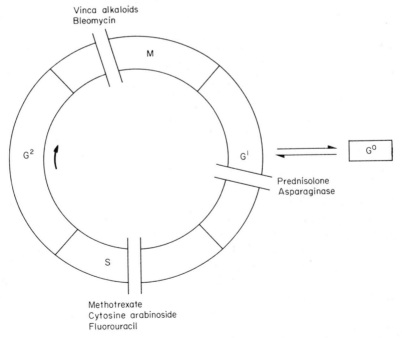

Fig. 4.2. Sites of action in the cell cycle of some phase-specific drugs.

The concept of phase specificity has had considerable therapeutic implications, particularly in combination regimens. The theories of 'synchronisation', i.e. bringing all dividing tumour cells in the cell cycle to the same phase at the same time then treating with a phase-specific drug, and of 'recruitment', i.e. destroying all dividing cells by means of a phase specific drug thus drawing resting tumour cells from G° into cycle for subsequent therapeutic attack, have received much attention. These ideas have so far proved more attractive in theory than in practice.

Single agent chemotherapy

Traditionally cytotoxic drugs were given singly in relatively low doses, often continuously, until tumour response was obtained. Although with our new found knowledge of cell cycle kinetics this approach is somewhat illogical, it is still the best form of therapy for some tumours.

Combination chemotherapy

Using cytotoxic drugs in combinations gives three major advantages:
1 Drugs of known effectiveness in treating a particular tumour, but with different actions as single agents, can be used with synergistic effects.
2 Drugs of different toxicities can be used to avoid cumulative adverse effects.
3 Using more than one drug in a regimen lessens the chance of resistance to the chemotherapy regimen.

Combination chemotherapy is usually given in 'pulses' at 3–4-week intervals to allow bone marrow recovery (Fig. 4.3).

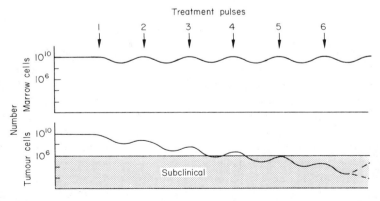

Fig. 4.3. Effects of pulsed chemotherapy on tumour and bone marrow cells.

In tumours with more cells in cycle (i.e. a larger growth fraction) than a normal tissue such as bone marrow, relatively more tumour cells than normal cells are killed with each treatment pulse and recovery of the tumour cell population is not complete before the next onslaught of chemotherapy. Also, the tumour cells are probably cycling more slowly and repairing less efficiently than normal cells; thus the pulse/kill effect is enhanced further.

High-dose chemotherapy

The realisation that the growth fraction of bone marrow cells (about 20%) is less than that of actively growing tumours and that it takes several days for resting marrow cells to come into cycle, has encouraged the use of high doses of pulsed chemotherapy given over a period of less than 24 hours in the knowledge that, provided the marrow is behaving normally, never more than a quarter is at risk.

Resistance

The development of resistance is a complex phenomenon usually involving the development of alternative pathways of DNA synthesis and division. It is a particular problem when single agents are used.

One explanation (suggested in the so-called Goldie–Coldman hypothesis) is that as tumours proliferate the malignant cells tend to mutate towards resistance to drugs never encountered. That is, the more tumour cells there are present, the greater the chance of their being resistant clones of cells. One approach to circumvent this possibility is the use of several drugs, together or in regimens, where combinations of non-cross-resistant drugs are used in alternating cycles of treatment.

Duration of therapy

The cytotoxic effects of drugs on tumour cells follow first order kinetics, so that for a given treatment the proportional reduction in tumour size is constant and not the number of cells killed in each treatment. Also we have seen earlier that the growth of the tumour is not linear; the same is true of the regression with treatment. If a tumour is chemosensitive then the number of cells will soon fall from being clinically evident (10^9–10^{12}) to clinically undetectable ($< 10^8$), but obviously many further courses of treatment will be necessary to eradicate the tumour cell population. This is not usually possible because of the increase in adverse effects on normal tissue with the increasing length of treatment. It is believed that the 'surveillance' system of the body can mop up tumour cells when their number is below a certain, as yet undefined, level. Nevertheless the question of when to stop chemotherapy is still unanswered, and the optimum duration of treatment is often decided on intuitive or empirical grounds, or by extrapolation from animal or *in vitro* cell kinetic studies.

Adverse effects

A summary of some of the more important adverse effects of drugs in common usage is given in Table 4.2. It will be seen that some adverse effects such as myelosuppression are seen with most drugs, whilst others are unique to individual drugs (e.g. cardiotoxicity with daunorubicin and doxorubicin). Cytotoxic chemotherapy should be given only by clinicians skilled in its use and with facilities for close monitoring of blood counts and disease status.

Common adverse effects

Complications at the injection site

This applies particularly to drugs administered by the intravenous route. Phlebitis, with or without thrombosis, of arm veins is common unless the drug is given where possible as an infusion or, when needed as a bolus, into a free running infusion or is carefully washed through with 20–50 ml of saline after injection. Leakage of cytotoxic drugs often gives local pain and induration; slow healing necrotic ulcers may result. Intramuscular drugs may give local pain and discomfort but this is usually temporary provided that the injection is given into the bulky muscle groups; occasionally the addition of a local anaesthetic (e.g. lignocaine) may be necessary. Care must be taken with intramuscular injections in patients with thrombocytopenia otherwise large haematomata may result.

Myelosuppression and immunosuppression

The patient with widespread malignant disease may have suppression of bone marrow and the lymphoreticular system before treatment is started. Cytotoxic chemotherapy may worsen the situation in such cases, unless the tumour burden decreases quickly with consequent improvement in the patient's general condition and resolution of tumour immunosuppressive effects. Great caution is therefore needed to avoid the possibility of overwhelming infection; regular checking of the blood count is vital and any infection must be treated early and aggressively. If possible marrow-sparing cytotoxic drugs (e.g. bleomycin and vincristine) should be considered. Protected (sterile) environments may be necessary in cases where cytotoxic

Table 4.2. Some adverse effects of commonly used cytotoxic drugs.

	Gut	Skin & mucosa	Hair	Phlebitis & necrosis	Lung	Heart	CNS & nerves	Liver	Urological	Marrow & immunity
ALKYLATING AGENTS										
Mustine	++	+	+	++	±		±			+++
Cyclophosphamide	+	+	++	+	±	±			+	++
Ifosfamide	++		+	+					+++	++
Chlorambucil	+	+			±			+		++
Melphalan	+	±			±					++
Busulphan	+	+			+					++
Thiotepa	+	+	+					+		++
Nitrosoureas	+	±	+	+	±			+	+	++
ANTIMETABOLITES										
Methotrexate	+	++	±		±			+	+	++
Purine and Pyrimidine analogues	+	+	±		±			+	±	+
VINCA ALKALOIDS										
Vincristine	+		++	++			+++			±
Vinblastine	+		+	++			++			++
ANTIBIOTICS										
Actinomycin D	+	+	+	++						++
Daunorubicin	+		+++	++		+++				++
Doxorubicin	+	+	+++	++		++				++
Bleomycin	+	+++	+	+	+++					
Mitozantrone	±	±	±	+		+				++
OTHERS										
Asparaginase	++	++					+	+		
Procarbazine	++	+					+		+	++
Dacarbazine	++	+	+	++						++
Cisplatin	++						++		++	++
Hydroxyurea	+	++	±					+		++
Etoposide	+		++							++

chemotherapy leads to profound leucopenia, for example in the treatment of acute leukaemia. Granulocyte transfusion, though short lived, may help during such leucopenic crises. Haemorrhage as a complication of cytotoxic drug-induced thrombocytopenia is fortunately uncommon; when it does occur platelet transfusions may be life saving.

Anaemia is a more long-term complication of myelosuppression; blood transfusion should be given as required in this situation. Blood transfusion will also improve tissue oxygenation and consequently the effectiveness of therapy.

Autologous (same patient) bone marrow transplantation is now being tried, in specialist centres, in some situations (e.g. in resistant lymphoma, myeloma and in certain solid tumours). Bone marrow is taken from the patient and freeze-stored until after high-dose chemotherapy with or without whole body irradiation; the bone marrow being then reinfused. Theoretically, maximal tumour cell killing will be achieved and profound myelotoxicity problems avoided.

Anaemia, leucopenia or thrombocytopenia in the patient undergoing chemotherapy for cancer should not always be attributed to the treatment. They may also indicate some paraneoplastic effect of the tumour, or indeed bone marrow involvement by the tumour. Examination of the blood film, differential white blood cell count and bone marrow will usually give the answer.

One further possible consequence of either the genetic damage or of the prolonged immunosuppression caused by cytotoxic agents is the apparent increased incidence of second neoplasms. It is also possible of course that the patient with one cancer is constitutionally more likely to develop another.

Skin, hair and mucosal problems

As with other drugs skin rashes of various types are not uncommon with cytotoxic drugs; if severe the offending drug must be stopped. Mouth ulcers are uncomfortable for the patient and are a feature particularly of methotrexate, fluorouracil and bleomycin therapy. Analgesia and good oral hygiene are of paramount importance. Hyperpigmentation may accompany the long-term use of certain drugs (e.g. bleomycin and busulphan), and alopecia, due to the depression of hair follicle growth cells, is a distressing adverse effect seen with many drugs including cyclophosphamide and the antibiotics. There is no consistent way of avoiding this (though scalp freezing may be successful in some situations) and it is best to warn the patient of the possibility of hair loss before treatment, reassuring them that it is usually temporary and arranging for a suitable wig to be made for them.

Gastrointestinal side effects

Nausea and vomiting are common side effects on the day of cytotoxic treatment. There are psychological and physical elements to these symptoms, and anti-emetic drugs such as prochlorperazine, metoclopramide and nabilone give helpful relief. Occasionally the symptoms persist for several days, presumably as a result of toxicity to the rapidly dividing small bowel epithelial cells. Diarrhoea may also be a problem but fortunately fatal gut toxicity is extremely uncommon and symptomatic treatment is usually very effective.

Germinal cell effects

Fetal conception during cytotoxic chemotherapy will result in abortion of the embryo, or in gross congenital abnormalities in the fetus, or in production of a child with genetic defects which may cause trouble in later life or in successive generations. To avoid these risks of teratogenesis and mutagenesis, chemotherapy should be avoided during the first trimester of pregnancy and given only if absolutely necessary later in the pregnancy.

Infertility (partial or total) can occur with cytotoxic chemotherapy. In males treated with alkylating agents sterility is inevitable. In younger female patients fertility may recover, though they may experience early menopause. Sperm freeze-storage prior to chemotherapy should be considered in those who request this, bearing in mind that such patients are often sub-fertile at presentation by virtue of their disease. If fertility recovers the patient should be advised to avoid conception for at least a year after cessation of treatment. The mutagenic risks in children conceived of parents who have had chemotherapy have not as yet had time to become apparent.

Less frequent side effects

Heart

Cardiomyopathy, manifested in tachycardia, ECG changes or overt heart failure, is a dose-related adverse effect of daunorubicin and doxorubicin. Routine ECG monitoring is recommended and caution should be exercised in patients with impaired cardiac function.

Lungs

Diffuse alveolar damage which may progress to fatal pulmonary fibrosis is seen with certain cytotoxic drugs. The main offender is bleomycin where regular clinical, radiological and respiratory function assessments are vital, but busulphan and certain other alkylating agents have also been incriminated.

Liver

Hepatotoxicity is an occasional side effect of many drugs (e.g. methotrexate and other antimetabolites). It usually takes the form of hepatocellular damage and may manifest as disordered liver function tests or as overt jaundice. The differential diagnosis from disseminated cancer can be difficult and may necessitate percutaneous liver biopsy to elucidate the answer.

Kidneys

Nephrotoxicity is surprisingly uncommon with cytotoxic drugs—perhaps the most important offender is cisplatin where dose-related and cumulative renal toxicity is the main limiting factor in treatment. Haemorrhagic cystitis may occur after ifosfamide or high-dose cyclophosphamide—this is usually preventable with mesna (see p. 52).

Nervous system

Neurotoxicity (which may affect peripheral, autonomic and cranial nerves) is common with the vinca alkaloids, particularly vincristine. Regular symptomatic enquiry and neurological testing are necessary when these drugs are being used. Methotrexate may also be neurotoxic and cisplatin can be ototoxic.

Metabolic

A 'wasting' syndrome with hyperpigmentation superficially resembling Addison's disease but without biochemical abormalities, may be seen with busulphan.

Hyperuricaemia, due to a rapid breakdown of tumour tissue, is possible with cytotoxic treatment of some cancers, particularly leukaemias and lymphomas. If the pretreatment serum uric acid level is high or if rapid tumour breakdown is expected, treatment with allopurinol is vital to avoid renal failure.

Special precautions

Drug dosages are usually calculated on surface area values. In patients with impaired renal or hepatic function, the doses of certain drugs excreted by the kidney or metabolised and excreted by the liver will have to be reduced; this information must always be checked from the relevant drug data sheets.

Interactions are a common problem with all forms of drug therapy; cytotoxic chemotherapy is no exception. Drug absorption may be affected by altering gastric emptying, for example with antiemetics, or by changing gut flora with antibiotics. Protein binding of cytotoxics (e.g. methotrexate) may be altered by administration of 'displacing' drugs, such as aspirin. Certain cytotoxic agents are antagonistic rather than synergistic in their tumouricidal action (e.g. methotrexate and cytosine arabinoside). Allopurinol enhances the effect of mercaptopurine by inhibiting enzymes concerned in its breakdown. These are just a few examples of what is certain to be an increasing problem in cytotoxic chemotherapy.

Some antagonistic interactions can be useful. The best example is the prevention of prolonged drug toxicity from methotrexate by the administration of folinic acid. 'Folinic acid rescue', as it is called, involves giving folinic acid 24–28 hours after a high dose of methotrexate, mainly to avoid damage to normal bone marrow resting cells recruited into cycle.

Social effects

In the cytotoxic chemotherapy of patients with cancer the quality of their existence during the period of treatment is of considerable importance. Some patients feel so wretched during and after the treatment that they develop anxiety/depression symptoms, and a positive dislike of coming for treatment (chemophobia) is not uncommon. Positive reassurance and morale boosting is an important part of such a patient's treatment.

Nevertheless most chemotherapy schedules allow the patient who is responding to treatment to get back to work apart from on the day of treatment. Out-patient treatment is therefore preferable for the mobile wage earner or the housewife. The patient so treated can also remain in contact with his general practitioner and local health services and the cost of chemotherapy, an increasing burden on the health service budget, is also kept to a minimum. In the old or infirm patient, however, or one travelling long distances for treatment, overnight accommodation in the hospital may be appropriate.

Cancer chemotherapy—an overview

Outstanding successes have been seen with cytotoxic chemotherapy, for example in choriocarcinoma, leukaemia, lymphoma and teratoma. Many other tumours respond often or occasionally to chemotherapy (Fig. 4.4). Others, however, rarely respond; so there is no cause for complacency. Further advances will be seen with the advent of new drugs and of new combination regimens and also, most importantly, from the properly controlled trials of appropriate chemotherapy in selected tumours in large numbers of patients. The place for 'adjuvant chemotherapy', that is the early use of cytotoxic chemotherapy (immediately after surgery or radiotherapy) when the number of malignant cells is small and when the cells are potentially at their most vulnerable, must also be assessed; particularly since this form of treatment may well subject cancer-free patients to all the short and long-term adverse effects of the cytotoxic drugs administered.

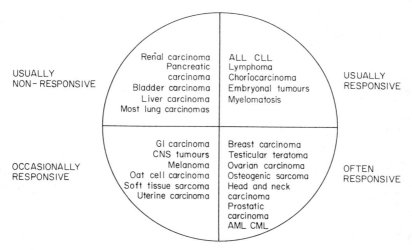

Fig. 4.4. Responsiveness of selected tumours to cytotoxic chemotherapy.

Chapter 5
Other Treatments

Surgery

The first therapeutic attempt is always the best, and sometimes the only, opportunity for cure of malignant disease. It is of the utmost importance, therefore, that the initial treatment is carefully considered. The known or likely extent of the disease, its expected response to the forms of treatment available, and its expected long-term behaviour all warrant assessment.

Surgery is the oldest method of treating malignant disease, but only in the last century has it become safe and effective with the greater appreciation of anatomical and physiological principles, the development of aseptic rather than antiseptic procedures, and the use of greatly improved anaesthetic agents and techniques.

Choice of treatment

It may be that surgery alone, or combined with radiotherapy and/or cytotoxic chemotherapy, offers the best chance of eradication of the disease. For some malignancies, particularly those in the 'radioresistant' group, surgery is usually the only form of radical treatment available; though with the development of new cytotoxic agents and regimens, these are becoming more important in the overall management of the disease.

Radical surgery

Radical surgery may result in little deformity or dysfunction, or alternatively significant physical and functional impairment may ensue. All surgical procedures carry some risk of operative morbidity and mortality, and in situations where a choice of treatments is available these must be carefully assessed. The general physical and medical state of the patient is also highly relevant to the form of management selected.

Tumour resection *en bloc* may offer the best opportunity for cure, where this is feasible without unacceptable morbidity or mortality. It may include removal of the regional lymphatic glands (block dissection) if these contain demonstrable deposits or there is a high risk of involvement.

Established procedures

Some radical surgical procedures have become well established. Radical mastectomy for early breast cancer was a standard operation for many decades, but more recently has become less popular, being replaced by local resection or simple mastectomy and postoperative radiotherapy. It was based on sound anatomical principles which required the removal of the whole breast, the pectoral muscles and the axillary lymph glands *en bloc*. The standard operation did not extend to removal of the internal mammary and supraclavicular lymph glands. It resulted in lymphoedema of the upper limb in a significant number of cases. The operation is associated with the name of Halstead.

Radical surgery for carcinoma of the uterine cervix was established by Wertheim; this operation involves removal of the uterus, a cuff of vagina, the fallopian tubes and ovaries, the broad ligaments and the pelvic lymph glands and lymphatics. This cannot be achieved entirely *en bloc* because of the need to carefully dissect out and preserve the ureters.

Abdominoperineal resection of the rectum for adenocarcinoma is also well established as a radical procedure. The involved section of bowel with a generous margin proximally, and the associated mesentery and lymph glands are removed up to the level of the inferior mesenteric artery. Partial colectomy with removal of the mesentery and the lymph glands draining the affected segment likewise is a standard operation for colonic cancer.

For operable gastric carcinoma, total gastrectomy again with removal of the draining lymph glands, is undertaken. In selected cases of thyroid cancer total thyroidectomy is appropriate. For operable involved lymph glands in one side of the neck from an ipsilateral primary tumour in the mouth area, *en bloc* dissection of the lymph glands, lymphatic channels, internal jugular vein and sternomastoid muscle offers a chance of cure.

Amputation of a limb may be the only method of eradicating a primary tumour in the radioresistant group (e.g. osteosarcoma, fibrosarcoma, synoviosarcoma), but this may have to be combined with cytotoxic chemotherapy in cases where early dissemination is likely or where established metastases are demonstrable.

Operative dissemination

Radical surgery for a localised tumour may not always prove curative. At operation tumour cells may be shed into the veins or lymphatic channels, and may disseminate to produce distant metastases, or may be seeded into the wound producing implantation deposits. Not all such cells survive, however; studies of venous blood and lymph draining from operation sites have shown the presence of tumour cells in up to 25% of cases, yet the incidence of overt metastases is much lower than this, and many of these cells must therefore be non-viable.

Surgery of access

Surgery may be an essential preliminary to further treatment. Selected cases of bladder carcinoma are treated by implantation of radioactive gold grains into the base of the tumour at open cystotomy.

Also it may be necessary to prepare a patient for definitive surgery to a tumour; a patient with intestinal obstruction from an operable carcinoma of the colon may require a colostomy as the first step followed later by resection of the tumour.

Adjuvant surgery

In situations where surgery alone is not potentially curative, it may nevertheless play a useful part in the management of the disease. Planned removal of a large primary tumour as a preliminary to radiotherapy and/or cytotoxic chemotherapy may be of great benefit by reducing the bulk of tumour to be treated. For example, a simple mastectomy for a breast carcinoma prior to radical radiotherapy to the breast area and proximal lymphatic drainage areas, reduces the chance of local tumour recurrence.

Total cystectomy for massive bleeding from an uncontrolled bladder carcinoma may be life-saving although not curative alone.

Removal of slow-growing and apparently solitary pulmonary metastases, for example from osteosarcoma or renal adenocarcinoma, may lead to an increased period of symptom-free survival.

Palliative surgery

Surgery may be of great value as palliation alone. A colostomy for lower large bowel obstruction from an advanced tumour may result in immediate relief of distressing symptoms. A tracheostomy for laryngeal obstruction may avert rapid death from asphyxia. A bypass operation for internal hydrocephalus caused by cerebral tumour may provide rapid relief of severe headaches, nausea and vomiting. Cordotomy or posterior rhyzotomy for intractable pain is another excellent example of palliative surgery.

Diagnostic surgery

Surgery is of paramount importance in obtaining tumour tissue for histopathological diagnosis; this may take the form of a simple operation like lymph gland excision biopsy, or of a more major procedure, as for example in the staging laparotomy of Hodgkin's disease.

Other surgical procedures

The surgical management of tumours in specific sites will be considered in more detail in the appropriate sections.

Immunotherapy

The possible roles of the immune response in cancer have been discussed (see Chapter 1). Immunotherapy in the patient with cancer aims at stimulating the cell mediated, humoral and phagocytic systems on the assumption that the normal immunological mechanisms have been unable to deal with the growing tumour. Evidence suggests that a powerful immunological reaction is necessary to destroy even a small number of malignant cells; the critical range of tumour cell acceptance or rejection seems to be 10^5–10^7 depending on the immunological state of the host. For malignant disease to become evident 10^8 cells are required; it follows that effective immunotherapy must depend on surgery, chemotherapy and radiotherapy for reducing the tumour burden to the minimum number of cells.

Table 5.1 summarises the methods of immunotherapy available.

Table 5.1. Immunotherapy in cancer.

PASSIVE	Administration of antibodies
ACTIVE	
Non-specific	BCG; *C. parvum*; levamisole; thymosin
Specific	Irradiated tumour cells; transfer factor
ADOPTIVE	
Non-specific	Unsensitised lymphoid cells
Specific	Sensitised lymphoid cells
LOCAL	Injection into tumour, e.g. BCG

Passive immunotherapy

Passive administration of antisera prepared against tumours has not proved successful in clinical practice and this treatment has the potential disadvantage of tumour enhancement; the antibodies, rather than destroying the tumour cells, may block the effective action of the lymphoid cells.

As we have seen, monoclonal antibodies against tumour antigens are providing new specific assays which may improve diagnosis and monitoring. Such antibodies are unlikely to kill cancer cells directly but may provide the 'magic bullet' to target cytotoxins to these cells.

Active non-specific immunisation

Active non-specific immunisation with BCG or *Corynebacterium parvum* stimulates all aspects of the immunological and phagocytic systems and in theory should enhance tumour cell destruction. Mathé in the late 1960s described good results with BCG therapy in acute lymphoblastic leukaemia, and many studies have since suggested possible benefit from both BCG and *C. parvum* therapy in combination with other forms of treatment. Many authorities however have found this form of immuno-therapy disappointing.

Levamisole, an effective synthetic anti-helminth with few toxic effects stimulates immune responses by unknown mechanisms. Stimulation is non-specific however and varies with dose and timing of administration. Recent reports suggest that it may be of adjuvant use in cancer therapy.

Thymosin, a thymic hormone of molecular weight 12 000 converts featureless null cells into T cells and has exciting possibilities in immuno-therapy; results in cancer therapy, however, are still awaited.

Active specific immunisation

Active specific immunisation has been attempted using irradiated tumour cells, and early results using irradiated leukaemic granulocytes in acute myeloid leukaemia were promising; however follow-up data have not been so convincing.

Transfer factor is a small molecular weight substance consisting of a short polypeptide chain joined to three or four RNA bases. It allows the specific transfer of cellular immunity by means of a cell-free non-antigenic extract. Its exact action is unknown but it undoubtedly improves T cell immunity and is concerned with the collaboration between T cells and other cells in the immunological system. It has already been used in the treatment of advanced melanoma and carcinoma, but its place in cancer therapy is far from firmly established.

Adoptive immunotherapy

Adoptive immunotherapy using unsensitised or sensitised lymphoid cells has proved of little help clinically, and of course in such treatment host v. graft or graft v. host reactions can be a major problem.

Local immunotherapy

Local immunotherapy, using injections of BCG or *C. parvum*, into the primary tumour or into secondary lymph node deposits may reduce tumour size but can be of only supportive, palliative value.

Summary

In summary immunostimulation holds exciting promise in the field of cancer therapy but has been bedevilled by the lack of controlled clinical trials. An example of this is in the wide publicity given to the antiviral agent interferon; this acts, probably via the immune system, as an anticancer agent but is as yet of unproven clinical value. Immunotherapy is not without adverse effects and can, at the present time, in no way replace the standard treatments of surgery, radiation and cytotoxic drugs; it should be given only as an adjuvant after the removal of the bulk of the tumour by those other treatments.

One major advance in immunotherapy (perhaps now better termed biological response modifier therapy) is the development of new molecular biological techniques. In this 'recombinant technology' large amounts of rare polypeptides involved in immune regulation can be produced by gene cloning and subsequent expression in tissue culture cells or microorganisms. Immune regulators, for example interferon and interleukins, produced in this way are presently being studied in clinical trials.

Endocrine therapy

The Scottish surgeon, Beatson, demonstrated in 1896 that oophorectomy can cause regression of metastatic breast carcinoma. It has since become apparent that the growth of some tumours is hormone dependent and that changing the balance of the hormonal environment can lead to regression of such tumours. A summary of the various endocrine procedures used in cancer therapy and of some of the side effects is given in Tables 5.2 and 5.3. Their more precise role will be defined in the appropriate chapters on treatment.

Hormone therapy is rarely curative, however, and often needs to be combined with other treatment modalities such as surgery, radiotherapy and chemotherapy. The recent recognition of the presence of hormonal receptors, particularly in breast cancer tissue, has made the use of endocrine treatment far less empirical, since detection of these receptors appears to be a reliable method of predicting hormonal responsiveness.

Table 5.2. Examples of endocrine therapy for cancer.

Tumour	Therapy
Breast	⎧ Oophorectomy
Premenopausal	⎪ (adrenalectomy,
Perimenopausal	⎨ hypophysectomy)
	⎪ Androgens
	⎪ Corticosteroids
	⎩ Anti-oestrogens
Postmenopausal	⎧ Oestrogens
	⎨ Anti-oestrogens
	⎩ Progestogens
Male	Orchidectomy, oestrogens
Prostate	Oestrogens, orchidectomy
Uterine body	Progestogens
Kidney	Progestogens
Haematological	Corticosteroids
Thyroid	Thyroxine

Table 5.3. Side effects of endocrine therapy.

OESTROGENS
Nausea, fluid retention, vaginal bleeding, feminisation, hypercalcaemia

ANDROGENS
Virilisation, cholestatic jaundice

ANTI-OESTROGENS
Nausea, skin rashes

PROGESTOGENS
Fluid retention, nausea

CORTICOSTEROIDS
Fluid retention, hypertension, diabetes, osteoporosis, Cushingoid features, immunosuppression

The role of steroids in cancer treatment deserves special consideration. Apart from their direct cytotoxic effect they have a role in the management of certain peripheral cancer effects. The physical and psychological well-being of a patient may be transiently improved, and hypercalcaemia and cerebral oedema (in association with brain metastases) may respond dramatically to prednisolone and dexamethasone respectively. Bone marrow suppression may occasionally respond to corticosteroids and/or androgens and it has been argued that steroids are myeloprotective. The only proven case for steroids in this situation however, is where an anaemia is of autoimmune haemolytic type. In all cases the considerable long-term side effects of treatment must be considered.

Chapter 6
Cancer of the Lung and Mediastinum

Primary lung cancer is essentially carcinoma of the bronchus. Occasionally carcinomas arise in the trachea, and malignant tumours of the pleura do occur.

Carcinoma of the bronchus

The bronchial tree is the commonest single site of cancer in man. Its incidence is increasing; the total number of deaths in England and Wales has increased five-fold over 35 years, thus:

1945 — 7 000
1955 — 17 000
1965 — 27 000
1975 — 30 000
1980 — 35 000

The incidence is higher in males than in females in the ratio of about 7 to 1, although this difference is decreasing as the incidence in females increases more rapidly than in males. It has been estimated that the incidence is increasing by 8% per decade in males and 50% in females. It is rare below the age of 25 years; the highest incidence is in the sixth decade in males and the seventh decade in females.

Lung cancer has been recognised as an industrial hazard for many years. Inhalation of asbestos dust is associated with pleural endothelioma and bronchial carcinoma; dust containing arsenicals, chromates and dichromates has a similar effect on the bronchial mucosa. Atmospheric pollution from industry and the internal combustion engine contribute. The cause *par excellance*, however, is tobacco smoking, particularly cigarettes.

Histology

The commonest histological types of cancer are shown in Table 6.1.

Carcinomas arise most commonly in the main bronchi or their first divisions, and most are therefore in the hilar regions. They may be mainly intrabronchial (papilliferous) or may infiltrate the bronchial wall; most

Table 6.1. Histological types of bronchial cancer.

COMMON TYPES

Squamous cell carcinoma (40-60% of lung cancers)—arising on areas of squamous
    metaplasia resulting from chronic irritation and the effects of carcinogens; much
    commoner in males
Undifferentiated carcinoma (about 30% of lung cancers)—mainly small cell (oat
    cell) tumours, but a few large cell lesions; also commoner in males
Adenocarcinoma (about 15% of lung cancers)—of equal incidence in the sexes

LESS COMMON TYPES

Cylindroma—which may involve the lower end of the trachea, and may be locally
    invasive
Alveolar cell carcinoma—which arises peripherally in the lung
Bronchial adenoma—usually benign
Carcinoid tumour—also usually benign

---

ultimately show both features and cause obstruction of the lumen. Primary
bronchial carcinoma is rarely bilateral.

Local spread is to adjacent structures—chest wall, mediastinum, pericardium, pleura and diaphragm. Lymphatic spread is via the mucosal,
peribronchial, pleural and perivascular vessels, with metastases to the
hilar, subcarinal, tracheobronchial, paratracheal and supraclavicular
nodes. Blood spread most commonly results in metastases to the bones,
brain, liver, suprarenal glands, kidney and the opposite lung. Spread by
bronchial aspiration has also been suggested.

Clinical features

The commonest symptoms are cough, dyspnoea and haemoptysis, similar
to those of bronchitis and bronchiectasis. Occasionally anorexia, fatigue, or
pyrexia of unknown origin are the presenting features. Some patients present with superior vena cava obstruction. Hoarseness, due to left recurrent
nerve palsy, or dysphagia due to pressure on the oesophagus from enlarged
mediastinal nodes may develop.

Horner's syndrome—ptosis, myosis, enophthalmos and anhydrosis, on
one side—will result from sympathetic ganglion involvement in the lower
neck. Tumours arising at the lung apex can invade the chest wall including
the ribs and branches of the brachial plexus, causing Pancoast's syndrome,
that is Horner's syndrome together with pain in the upper limb, wasting of
the small muscles of the hand and destructive areas in the upper two or
three ribs, on the affected side.

Hypertrophic pulmonary osteoarthropathy (HPOA) and digital clubbing may occur as paraneoplastic manifestations; the former presents as painful expansion of the lower ends of the radii and sometimes of the tibiae; clubbing occurring without HPOA is a suggestive but not diagnostic feature.

Other non-metastatic effects include cerebellar ataxia, peripheral neuropathy, and ectopic hormone secretion (see Chapter 16). In disseminated disease there may be symptoms related to metastases.

Investigations

In the investigation of bronchial cancer, radiology is of great value. Posteroanterior and lateral films of the chest are required, since some significant parts of the lungs cannot be clearly visualised on posteroanterior films alone. Tomography in the sagittal plane is helpful, and now computerised axial tomography is proving of immense value, particularly in the assessment of the mediastinum. Barium swallow may show oesophageal compression by node masses. Bronchoscopy, or sometimes mediastinoscopy, with biopsy is indicated where possible. Lung scans of ventilation and perfusion types can also be of value.

Treatment

It is generally accepted that the only potentially curative treatment of localised squamous carcinoma and adenocarcinoma is surgical excision—lobectomy or pneumonectomy as appropriate. This is possible in only about 4% of cases; in the remainder the disease is too advanced or operation is contraindicated by the patient's general condition, limited pulmonary reserve or coincidental disease.

Radical radiotherapy is applicable only to tumours which are surgically operable, but where surgery is contraindicated on the above grounds. A beam-directed technique is used and allowance for lung transmission is made where necessary.

Surgery is not appropriate in the management of undifferentiated small cell carcinomas (oat cell carcinomas). These tumours spread early to local lymph nodes, and disseminate early via the bloodstream, typically producing metastases in the brain, bones and liver. Radiotherapy is indicated to the mediastinum, hilar and supraclavicular areas; this treatment is often combined with irradiation of the brain and combination cytotoxic chemotherapy. One schedule of chemotherapy includes doxorubicin, fluorouracil and methotrexate (with folinic acid rescue) in pulsed courses. Alternatively, high-dose intravenous cyclophosphamide can be given with or without radiotherapy. Newer agents being studied in combination chemotherapy include ifosfamide (with mesna), etoposide and cisplatin.

Palliative irradiation may be very helpful in the treatment of superior vena cava obstruction, haemoptysis, dyspnoea due to lobar or lung collapse, and persistent cough. It is of less value in the treatment of mediastinal pain and oesophageal obstruction. Local treatment to bony metastases usually offers good pain relief. Brain irradiation for metastases is of value only for oat cell carcinoma deposits.

In the palliative treatment of squamous cell carcinomas bleomycin is of some value. The complication of lung fibrosis must be remembered, and respiratory function checked before each course, and further treatment withheld if this is significantly reduced. Large cell carcinomas have been treated palliatively with doxorubicin, cyclophosphamide and methotrexate in combination.

The management of locally advanced but asymptomatic disease is debatable. Some authorities argue that treatment is essentially palliative and that if there are no symptoms to palliate no treatment is required. Others argue that locally advanced disease will progress and produce symptoms sooner or later and that treatment to a smaller volume will be more effective than to a larger volume. In practice, each case must be considered individually.

Results

The results of treatment of lung cancer are very poor. About 80% of patients are dead within 1 year, and overall 5-year survival is about 5%. Pneumonectomy yields figures of about 25% at 5-years; operative mortality is 5–10%. Lobectomy gives about 30% 5-year survival, with operative mortality of 2–5%. Small peripheral tumours fare much the same—30% at 5 years. Radical radiotherapy shows 5-year survival in a mere 3–5% of cases.

Cancer of the trachea

This is rare. One series reported five cases over a 5-year period, during which 1600 cases of bronchial carcinoma were treated. It is commonest in the middle and lower thirds of the trachea. Most tumours are squamous cell carcinomas; occasionally cylindromas are reported. Radical surgery is rarely possible, and radiotherapy yields poor results.

The rarity of cancer of the trachea is interesting, considering its relatively high incidence in the respiratory tract above (the larynx) and very high incidence below (in the bronchi).

Tumours of the pleura

Primary tumours of the pleura are uncommon. Most frequent are localised fibromas, which are resectable, and diffuse endotheliomas (mesotheliomas) some of which are malignant, and which may be difficult to treat. In the latter tumours, local palliative radiotherapy may be needed for pain relief. Cytotoxic chemotherapy is of little value. Results of treatment are poor.

Mediastinal tumours

Primary tumours of the mediastinum are uncommon; about one-third are malignant. They are listed in Table 6.2.

Dermoids

Dermoids (teratomas) occur predominantly in the 10–30-year age group. Almost invariably they arise in the anterior mediastinum, usually in front of the pericardium and great vessels. Usually they contain tissues from all three layers of the embryo, mainly skin, hair, sebaceous material, and glandular tissue. Most are benign, but a few are malignant most commonly in their squamous epithelial elements.

Neurogenic tumours

Neurogenic tumours usually arise in the posterior mediastinum. They can vary greatly in size, and can weigh as much as 1 kg. If they arise from nerve elements near an intervertebral foramen the typical dumb-bell tumour results, with part inside the spinal canal and part outside, and with enlargement of the foramen demonstrable radiologically; the best example of this is in multiple neurofibromatosis (von Recklinghausen's disease).

Neuroblastomas occur almost exclusively in childhood. They are highly radiosensitive. Some show areas of well differentiated ganglioneuroma,

Table 6.2. Mediastinal tumours.

DERMOID CYSTS (teratomas)—the commonest

NEUROGENIC TUMOURS
(a) Neuroblastoma, ganglioneuroma, pheochromocytoma—arising from nerve cells of the sympathetic system
(b) Neurilemmoma, neurosarcoma, neurofibroma—arising from nerve sheaths

THYMOMA

RARE TUMOURS, such as lipoma and liposarcoma, paraganglioma, haemangioma, tumours similar histologically to choriocarcinoma, benign and malignant mesenchymal tumours of the heart, mesothelioma of the pericardium (usually malignant) and leiomysarcoma of the great vessels

---

and have a better prognosis. Occasionally, spontaneous transformation from neuroblastoma to ganglioneuroma occurs (see Chapter 12).

Thymoma

Thymomas account for about 10% of mediastinal tumours. Almost invariably they arise in the anterior mediastinum. They may be true neoplasms or simple hypertrophy of the thymic tissues. They are commonest in middle age. About 10% are benign cysts; about 30% are invasive. Four histological types are described: lymphocytic, epithelial, mixed, and spindle-celled. Occasionally the histological appearance resembles seminoma, and occasionally there is a granulomatous appearance which has been regarded as primary thymic Hodgkin's disease. Some are associated with myasthenia gravis; 10% of patients with this condition have a thymoma, and 50% of patients with a thymoma have myasthenia gravis.

Clinical features

Malignant mediastinal tumours may metastasise to local lymph nodes, to the liver, lungs, and brain, and to other sites rarely. They infiltrate locally, and early symptoms are due to this. Retrosternal pain, dyspnoea and cough are common in anterior mediastinal tumours; cough, pain from brachial plexus or nerve root involvement, hoarseness from left recurrent laryngeal nerve involvement, and dyspnoea due to pleural effusion are common in posterior mediastinal tumours. Radiologically, paradoxical movements of the diaphragm may indicate phrenic nerve paralysis, and oesophageal compression may be demonstrable. Heart tumours may produce gradually increasing congestive heart failure, or sudden death.

Benign tumours may be large before producing any symptoms or signs. About one-third are diagnosed on routine radiology.

Tumours which have produced symptoms for over 1 year are usually benign. Pain or the signs of superior vena cava obstruction usually indicate a malignant tumour. The rare choriocarcinoma will be associated with high levels of beta-HCG in the blood and urine, and the rare malignant teratoma may produce raised levels of alpha-fetoprotein in the blood. Pheochromocytoma may produce episodes of hypertension. Neuroblastoma will show increased urinary output of catecholamine breakdown products.

Radiology may be helpful; teratomas may contain demonstrable calcification or rudimentary teeth, and neurogenic tumours may enlarge the intervertebral foramina or produce local absorption of vertebral bodies or ribs. The only basis for an exact diagnosis is biopsy.

Management

In management, thoracotomy should be considered for diagnosis and if possible for removal of the tumour. Operative mortality, in competent hands, is surprisingly low. Radiotherapy may be indicated for the primary tumour or for residue after surgery. It may be curative in neuroblastoma and thymoma, and it may achieve long-term control in malignant teratoma (though this is now often treated with chemotherapy). Combination cytotoxic chemotherapy may be needed for neuroblastoma—cyclophosphamide with vincristine and doxorubicin has proved of value (see Chapter 12).

Radiation side effects include dysphagia and irritant cough during and immediately after treatment, and occasionally the symptoms of pulmonary fibrosis and pericardial fibrosis occur later.

Results

The results of treatment depend upon the type of tumour. Benign tumours can usually be excised and do well. Thymomas vary in their response, but overall 5-year survival of 20% is reported for malignant types. For neuroblastoma 60% 3-year survival is claimed. For other tumours, the numbers treated are too small to allow for accurate assessment.

Other mediastinal tumours

Malignant lymphatic involvement is the commonest cause of mediastinal tumour; malignant lymphoma and secondary carcinoma (e.g. from bronchus) are the usual offenders. The management of these tumours is discussed under the appropriate headings.

Chapter 7
Breast Cancer

The breast is the commonest site of malignant disease in women; and breast malignancy is the commonest cause of death in women in the age group 40–44 years. Its incidence increases with age, being uncommon below the age of 30, and its behaviour varies from slowly progressive to rapidly progressive disease despite all forms of treatment.

Aetiology

The aetiology of human breast cancer is not known; there is a familial tendency, but the single most important factor is hormone status. It is predominantly a disease of women (100 : 1 female to male ratio), occuring less frequently with multiple pregnancy, with prolonged breast feeding and with early gonadal ablation, and it may be responsive to various hormonal treatments. Cystic breast disease (fibroadenosis) and higher social class also increase the risk of breast cancer.

Pathology

Pathologically the majority of breast cancers are infiltrating duct cell adenocarcinomas with varying degrees of fibrous tissue reaction. If the fibrous reaction is pronounced the term schirrous carcinoma is used. Other adenocarcinomas include the lobular, medullary, colloid, tubular, cribriform and papillary variants, and a very small proportion of breast cancers is composed of sarcomas, lymphomas and various metastatic carcinomas.

It is likely that breast cancer is often a systemic disease at the time of presentation. Overt metastasis occurs by local infiltration to skin and opposite breast, by lymphatics to regional lymph nodes (axillary, supraclavicular fossa and internal mammary) and by bloodstream to bone, lungs, liver and brain. Bone secondaries are present in over half of patients with disseminated disease. Hypercalcemia is common in breast cancer usually as a result of overt or microscopic bone disease, probably in association with local or systemic production of some osteolytic ectopic substance; oestrogen therapy may exacerbate the hypercalcemia of breast carcinoma.

Clinical presentation

Clinical presentation is most often by detection by the patient of a breast lump or other abnormality of the breast or its overlying skin. Sometimes the presentation is by metastasis, particularly to bone where both osteolytic and osteoblastic deposits may be found. Other presentations (such as pleural effusion, brain metastases and hypercalcemia) are far less common.

Examination of the breast area will delineate the position and extent of the tumour, its fixation and involvement of lymph nodes, particularly in the axilla. Skin involvement is not uncommon; oedema of the skin (giving the classical *peau d'orange* appearance) and eczematous patches over the nipple and immediately surrounding skin (Paget's disease) usually indicate an intraduct carcinoma; local infiltration with ulceration, erythema and venous engorgement are also seen. Acute inflammation of the breast is seen with so-called 'inflammatory carcinoma', and local skin lymphatics may be permeated leading to skin nodularity, so-called *cancer-en-cuirasse*.

Diagnosis

Differential diagnosis of smaller breast lesions can be difficult, particularly in the presence of fibroadenosis. Mammography may be helpful, but histological verification is mandatory either by needle biopsy or by excision of the suspected lump, often with frozen section histology (see later).

If the diagnosis is confirmed some sort of staging of the disease is vital. Several staging systems have been advocated; the TNM (tumour, node, metastasis) system is gradually gaining acceptance, but the simplest system is to grade the disease as local, that is confined to the breast, regional, when the axillary nodes are involved, or distant, when there is evidence of wider spread metastases. A clinical staging procedure popular in the UK is summarised in Table 7.1.

It has already been stated that the disease may be occultly widespread at presentation. However haematological, biochemical, radiological (chest

Table 7.1. Clinical staging of breast carcinoma.

Stage 1 Mobile tumour (< 5 cm diameter) with or without *local* skin involvement

Stage 2 As above plus palpable mobile ipsilateral axillary nodes

Stage 3 Tumour > 5 cm diameter with involvement of underlying muscle or of skin wide of the tumour or axillary node fixation

Stage 4 Presence of distant metastases (other than axillary nodes)

---

and skeletal survey) and radioisotopic bone scanning investigations should be done to get the maximum amount of information as to the degree of overt spread.

Hormone receptor status

Hormone receptor status now plays an important part in the preliminary assessment of patients with breast cancer. It is now known that the hormone receptor content of tumours provides an index of their hormone responsiveness. As with other hormone-sensitive tissues the essential first step in the response of these tumours is the binding of the hormone to the receptor protein in the target cell cytoplasm or on the cell membrane. The assay of specific steroid receptor proteins is possible by utilising the receptor's ability to bind tightly to tritium labelled steroids. Oestrogen receptors are present in over 60% of tumours, progesterone receptors in over 30%, and androgen receptors in over 20%. It seems likely that the finding of oestrogen or of oestrogen and progesterone receptor tissue in breast cancer indicates that the tumour will be responsive to hormonal therapy and indeed may have an altogether better prognosis.

Management

The management of breast carcinoma provides a major challenge. Many forms of treatment in numerous combinations have been used (Table 7.2), and it is therefore difficult to generalise as regards overall management; nevertheless some guidelines are available. A simplified scheme for conventional management in breast cancer is given in Fig. 7.1.

After detailed assessment of the patient's status most authorities proceed to some form of mastectomy; the mutilating major procedure of radical mastectomy is not now generally thought necessary. Some authorities rely on local excision of the tumour (lumpectomy) and follow this by some form of adjuvant therapy. At operation where the diagnosis of cancer is in doubt frozen section histology should give the answer. At mastectomy axillary nodes may be biopsied and later histologically examined.

Subsequent management depends on the information so far accumulated. Certain prognostic factors are important (Table 7.3).

Lesions of large size are more likely to be associated with metastasis. Inner quadrant, skin and pectoral muscle involving lesions are likely to recur locally. Prognosis is good when no axillary nodes are involved, intermediate when 1–4 nodes are involved and poor when more than four nodes are involved. Axillary node involvement is less frequent with medullary, colloid and papillary adenocarcinomas and prognosis consequently better.

Table 7.2. Management of breast cancer.

SURGERY
Excision biopsy
Simple mastectomy
Total mastectomy
(Radical mastectomy)

RADIOTHERAPY
Postoperative
(Preoperative)
Palliative

ENDOCRINE
Ovarian ablation
(Adrenalectomy)
(Pituitary ablation)
Corticosteroids   } Selected pre-
(Aminoglutethimide)   and perimenopausal
Androgens   patients
Tamoxifen

Oestrogens
Tamoxifen   } Selected postmenopausal
Progestogens   patients

CYTOTOXIC CHEMOTHERAPY
(Adjuvant early)
Disseminated disease—selected patients

Widely metastatic disease is obviously of worse prognosis than local or regional disease. The prognostic indications of hormone receptor status have already been discussed.

Radiotherapy

Postoperative radiation therapy to the breast and proximal lymphatic drainage areas may be appropriate when the breast lesion is large and fixed, particularly in the inner quadrant, when the axillary nodes are involved and when there is evidence of lymphatic permeation. Radical postoperative radiotherapy is directed to the chest wall anteriorly and laterally, and to the axillary, supraclavicular and internal mammary lymph node areas on the affected side. It may not be needed where the initial lesion is a completely excised, small, mobile tumour free of histological features of infiltration or lymphatic spread. This form of treatment is also not appropriate when widespread disease is evident.

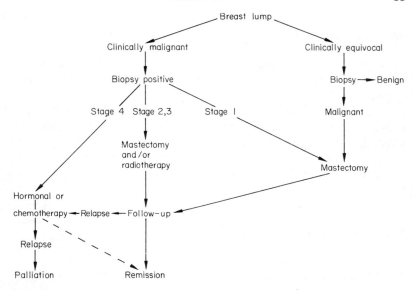

Fig. 7.1. Simplified conventional management scheme for breast carcinoma.

Table 7.3. Prognostic factors in breast cancer.

1 Size and position of the lesion
2 Fixation and infiltration of the lesion
3 Axillary node status
4 Histology
5 Stage of the disease
6 Hormone receptor status

Adjuvant postoperative irradiation reduces the incidence of local recurrence but does not increase survival. Nevertheless such treatment may result in many years of normal or near normal life; in many patients with occult metastasis at presentation it may be a long time before such spread produces symptoms and becomes manifest.

Some authorities prefer preoperative radiotherapy to postoperative treatment. It is argued that the local blood supply to the tissues is better before than after surgery, so that improved tumour responses and less marked radiation reactions result. Also, any tumour cells seeded at operation will be of reduced viability, thus decreasing the chances of local residual deposits or distant metastases. Others argue that after radiotherapy postoperative healing may be delayed. In general, preoperative treatment is less commonly used than postoperative treatment.

For the treatment of inoperable, widespread or recurrent disease cyto-toxic chemotherapy or hormonal therapy are appropriate, though radiotherapy has an important place in palliation in such patients. It will reduce the local tumour mass, healing ulceration and controlling bleeding and discharge. For the immediate management of local bone metastases it can be very effective in controlling pain, reducing the tumour mass and en-couraging healing of the bone; it may forestall the occurrence of pathological fractures in long bones or the development of paraplegia from spinal deposits. For intracranial metastases it may control the headaches, nausea and vomiting of raised intracranial pressure, especially in combi-nation with dexamethasone therapy. In this situation however it has the disadvantage of causing hair loss.

Endocrine therapy

The choice of hormonal or cytotoxic chemotherapy for advanced disease depends on the menstrual and hormone receptor status of the patient. Overall about one-third of breast cancers are hormone responsive; this figure can be improved to over a half by judicious selection. In hormone receptor positive patients hormonal manipulation is more appropriate, but even in those patients who are receptor negative or of unknown status en-docrine therapy may still be beneficial.

The premenopausal patient

In the premenopausal patient ovarian ablation (oophorectomy or less often ovarian irradiation) is usually first undertaken. Best responses are seen in the age group 35–45 years and where the disease has been slowly pro-gressive. Those who show a response have a better chance of also respond-ing to other endocrine procedures. Oophorectomy may be followed by bilateral adrenalectomy or ablation of the pituitary gland (as by yttrium-90 implant) though these procedures have fallen into disuse in many centres. The so-called medical adrenalectomy, by the administration of exogenous corticosteroid drugs or aminoglutethimide to suppress endogenous steroid synthesis, still has a place in management. In the premenopausal patient androgens (e.g. fluoxymesterone) may also be given, though their virilising side effects may be unwelcome. More often these days tamoxifen, an anti-oestrogenic compound without androgenic properties which competes with oestrogen for binding sites in target organs, is given. It is relatively free of side effects and the proportion of patients with breast cancer who respond to tamoxifen is similar to that seen with other hormones.

The postmenopausal patient

In patients more than 5 years postmenopausal, particularly when hormone receptor positive, hormonal therapy (e.g. with tamoxifen or less often ethinyloestradiol) is appropriate; good responses are seen particularly in older patients with predominantly skin or lymph node metastases.

The perimenopausal patient

Perimenopausal patients (from the menopause to 5 years following this) are difficult to manage, though ovarian ablation is occasionally effective, particularly in receptor positive patients. However, tamoxifen is usually considered as a first-line measure in perimenopausal patients with locally or generally advanced disease.

Other 'hormone' therapies to be considered as second or third-line measures, particularly in the postmenopausal patient, are progestogens (e.g. medroxyprogesterone, megesterol) and aminoglutethimide, which acts as an inhibitor of adrenal steroid production and also inhibits conversion of androgens to oestrogens in peripheral tissues.

All forms of hormone therapy may cause an initial transient 'flare' or exacerbation of the disease; hypercalcaemia is the most notable manifestation of this flare.

Chemotherapy

Cytotoxic chemotherapy may be appropriate for those patients who are hormone receptor negative or who are resistant to hormone therapy. With combination regimens about one-half of such patients will show response to treatment. Side effects are inevitable and the principles of administration and combination (see Chapter 4) are important to ensure maximum tumoricidal effect with minimum normal tissue disturbance. Chemotherapy may also be appropriate for pre- and perimenopausal patients with unknown hormone receptor status and rapidly progressive disease where the disease free interval is less than 2 years; for slowly progressive disease hormonal procedures may be tried first. In postmenopausal patients with unknown receptor status oestrogens or tamoxifen may still give good responses.

The choice of drugs and manner of administration to get the best results in breast cancer is not yet certain; parenteral combination chemotherapy is probably best, and regimens containing two or more of doxorubicin, cyclophosphamide, vinca alkaloid, methotrexate and fluorouracil seem to be giving the most promising results.

The case for early adjuvant cytotoxic chemotherapy (that is, breast surgery immediately followed by a cytotoxic chemotherapy regimen) is not yet practically proven. The theory is that early chemotherapy will deal with occult distant metastases known to be present in many patients at the time of presentation, on the argument that the smaller the number of active tumour cells to be treated the greater the chance of eradicating them. In practice this could mean subjecting potentially cured women to toxic therapy, and the long-term results of ongoing controlled trials on this subject are awaited with interest; certainly preliminary results indicate modestly improved relapse-free survival in certain pre-menopausal patients.

Tamoxifen may also have a role as early adjuvant therapy, particularly in postmenopausal patients.

Prognosis

Prognosis is difficult to assess in breast cancer because the natural history of the disease is not known for certain. Undoubtedly some patients are cured by local treatment alone but the overall mortality is about 50% at 5–6 years, the death rate being greatest in the first 3 years. The majority of women with breast cancer still die from the disease or its complications.

The results of large controlled trials suggest that the prognosis is improving with newer schemes of management, but are again difficult to interpret because of the long natural history of the disease.

Screening

Screening for breast cancer is possible using techniques such as clinical examination, mammography and thermography. Cancer education programmes are encouraging the technique of self-examination of the breast. Hopefully these procedures will result in the detection of early cancers amenable to treatment; their great cost however, particularly with screening programmes, limits their application in a financially constrained health service.

Male breast cancer

Male breast cancer is uncommon but occurs with increased frequency in Klinefelter's syndrome. The pathology and clinical pattern is similar to that for female breast cancer and the appropriate management by surgery, endocrine manipulation (particularly orchidectomy), radiotherapy or chemotherapy can produce useful sustained remissions.

Chapter 8
Alimentary Tract Cancer

The upper alimentary tract above the pharyngo-oesophageal junction is considered in Chapter 9; the remainder can be divided into sections:

1 Oesophagus.
2 Stomach.
3 Liver, pancreas and gall bladder.
4 Duodenum, jejunum and ileum.
5 Caecum, colon, and rectum.
6 Anal canal and anus.

Oesophagus

Malignant tumours of the oesophagus represent about 5% of all cancers, and occur mainly in later life. They are commoner in males than in females. The majority are squamous cell carcinomas, arising in the stratified epithelium of the upper and middle thirds of the oesophagus; adenocarcinomas arise at the lower end in gastric-type mucosa which can extend a short distance up into the oesophagus.

Local infiltration occurs early with both circumferential and longitudinal spread; the former results in stenosis, and by virtue of the latter the upper and lower limits of a tumour may extend well beyond those demonstrable by oesophagoscopy or radiology. Lymphatic spread also occurs early to mediastinal, neck and upper abdominal nodes, and is present in about 50% of tumours 5 cm or more in length.

Symptoms

The main symptom is dysphagia, initially for solids and later for fluids also. Later, weight loss occurs. The level of the dysphagia can sometimes be fairly well localised by the patient. Tumours arise most often at one of the areas of partial natural narrowing of the oesophagus, namely the pharyngo-oesophageal junction (40%), the junction of upper and middle thirds where it is crossed by the left main bronchus (40%), and at the lower end where the oesophagus passes through the diaphragm (20%).

89

Investigations

The most valuable investigations are endoscopy (oesophagoscopy) and radiology (barium swallow). At oesophagoscopy a biopsy can be taken and the lumen dilated if necessary.

Management

Management depends on the level of the tumour. The upper third of the oesophagus is closely related to other vital structures in the mediastinum, and surgical clearance and reconstruction is very difficult or impossible. High-dose radiotherapy is indicated for lesions not more than 5 cm long; more extensive lesions will have infiltrated widely and produced lymph node metastases, and are beyond radical treatment. Middle third lesions are more accessible by the lateral transthoracic approach, and early tumours are resectable. For radiotherapy, the same criteria apply as for upper third tumours. Lower third tumours are the most accessible, by a combined thoracic and abdominal route; excision is the only potentially curative treatment, as adenocarcinomas are radioresistant.

Preoperative radiotherapy is advocated by some authorities, but has limited applications, and its role has not been established.

Palliative radiotherapy is rarely of value; tumours beyond radical treatment are usually far advanced and symptomatic improvement is unlikely. Better palliation can be achieved, with less upset, by the insertion of a plastic tube to maintain a lumen (Mousseau–Barbin or Celestin type).

Results

Results are disappointing; overall figures quoted are about 20% 5-year survival for upper third tumours, about 6% for middle third, and about 15% for lower third.

Stomach

Gastric cancer is one of the commonest malignancies of western civilisation, having been overtaken in males only recently by bronchial cancer. Its highest incidence is in the sixth decade, it is twice as common in males than females, and it is commonest in the higher social classes. It occurs three times more frequently in the absence of normal gastric secretion (achlorhydria). It is said that long-standing gastric ulcers can undergo malignant changes, but this is not proven.

The vast majority of cancers are adenocarcinomas; others include lymphoma, leiomyosarcoma and carcinoid tumours, but the latter two are rarities. Adenocarcinoma may be diffuse and infiltrating, fungating or ulcerated. The diffuse variety produces the classical 'leather bottle stomach'. Local extension leads to invasion of adjacent structures. Lymphatic spread to local nodes occurs early; later, deposits in the supraclavicular nodes, especially on the left (Troisier's sign), become evident. Spread to the liver via the portal system is common. Transcoelomic spread results in deposits on the pelvic peritoneum and on the ovaries, and often on both (Krukenberg tumours).

Symptoms

Early symptoms are vague. Appetite gradually deteriorates, and weight is slowly lost. Irregular mild upper abdominal discomfort or pain may be dismissed as 'indigestion'. Haematemesis, or signs of pyloric obstruction may draw attention to the lesion. Anaemia is not uncommon. Later, abdominal swelling due to ascites may develop.

Investigations

Investigations include barium meal examination, which may show an irregular filling defect or a rigid stomach wall, and gastroscopy which also allows a biopsy to be taken.

Treatment

The only radical treatment available is surgical excision of the stomach (gastrectomy) and adjacent lymph node groups. Radiotherapy has nothing to offer, either as radical or palliative treatment. Recently, useful palliation has been claimed for combination cytotoxic therapy, using fluorouracil, doxorubicin and carmustine.

Results

The overall results of surgery are about 25% 5-year survival. However, many tumours are inoperable when diagnosed, and at present the only hope of improving results lies in earlier diagnosis.

Liver, pancreas and gall bladder

Malignant disease of these organs accounts for as many deaths as gastric cancer in males and as breast cancer in females.

The liver

Primary malignancy of the liver (hepatoma) is uncommon, although its incidence is four times higher in males than in females, and higher in oriental and dark-skinned races. In more than half the cases, it is associated with cirrhosis of the liver. The hepatitis B virus and mould toxins are known aetiological factors. A form termed hepatoblastoma occurs in children.

Symptoms

The main symptoms and signs are malaise, local pain and obstructive jaundice; later, a mass may be palpable. In many cases, the level of serum alpha-fetoprotein is raised, and this is a useful marker for diagnosis and the monitoring of response to treatment.

Treatment

Treatment is essentially surgical; results are poor with less than 1% surviving 5 years. Intra-arterial cytotoxic chemotherapy has its advocates, but responses are poor and inconsistent, and associated upset can be severe.

The pancreas

Adenocarcinoma of the pancreas is a disease of later life. It affects males more frequently than females, and it arises more often in the head of the organ than in the tail, but only in proportion to the amount of tissue in each part. Progress of the tumour is insidious. Regional lymph node involvement and liver deposits occur early, and bone and lung metastases are not uncommon. Jaundice, due to bile duct obstruction, is the cardinal sign, but usually indicates advanced disease.

Treatment

Treatment again is surgical; these tumours are resistant to radiotherapy and cytotoxic chemotherapy. Operability rates are low and 5-year survival figures quoted are less than 1%. Palliative cholecystoduodenostomy may be of temporary benefit.

The gall bladder

Malignancy of the gall bladder and extrahepatic bile ducts is also a disease of later life. In contrast to primary liver cancer, it is almost four times as common in females as in males. Calculi are present in a high proportion of cases, figures as high as 100% being quoted. The majority of lesions are adenocarcinomas, but about 10% are squamous cell carcinomas.

Symptoms

Symptoms usually are vague until a late stage of the disease, and an exact diagnosis without laparotomy may be difficult or impossible. Cholecysto-graphic findings may be indefinite.

Treatment

Radical treatment is often impossible because of local invasion, lymph node metastases, seedling deposits along the biliary tract, and distant metastases, the latter not infrequently in the lungs or bones. Radiotherapy and cytotoxic chemotherapy are of no value. Palliative treatment, apart from sedatives and analgesics, likewise has nothing to offer. With the exception of very early tumours discovered incidentally at cholecystec-tomy, 5-year survival figures are a mere 0–2%.

The close association between gallstones and gall bladder cancer has been advanced as a strong argument in favour of cholecystectomy in all cases of gallstones.

Duodenum, jejunum and ileum

Malignant disease of these organs is rare. The only one warranting atten-tion here is lymphoma, which occasionally arises in the Peyer's patches. Usually it is of non-Hodgkin's type. It presents as vague bowel upset, as obstruction or as a malabsorption syndrome. It is managed in the same way as lymphoma arising in other areas of lymphoid tissue, and the prognosis is similar (about 45% well at 5 years, overall).

Small bowel carcinoid tumours are discussed in Chapter 16.

Caecum, colon and rectum

Cancer of the large bowel is common, and in white races accounts for more deaths than any other form of malignant disease. It occurs mainly in mid-dle and old age, and affects males and females equally. The principal sites are the caecum and ascending colon (15%), rectosigmoid region (40%) and rectum (35%). Thus, about three-quarters of tumours arise within access of sigmoidoscopy.

Predisposing factors

Predisposing factors include single or multiple polyps, especially familial polyposis, and long-standing ulcerative colitis. Sluggish bowel movement has been incriminated, particularly in developed countries where the diet is low in residue and possibly high in carcinogens from food additives and preservatives.

Symptoms

Almost all large bowel cancers are adenocarcinomas. They may be of exophytic or ulcerative, infiltrative types. Blood and mucus in the faeces is a common presenting symptom; later, evidence of subacute or acute intestinal obstruction supervenes, and alternating constipation and diarrhoea is classical. Tumour spread is via the lymphatics and the bloodstream; blood-borne metastases may reach the liver directly by the portal system.

Investigations

Investigations include sigmoidoscopy (or colonoscopy) and biopsy for accessible tumours, and barium enema examination. The latter can be supplemented by air insufflation to obtain double contrast radiographs.

Treatment

Caecal and colonic adenocarcinomas are radioresistant, and attempts at radical radiotherapy are fraught with problems, such as ulceration of the bowel wall, perforation and obstruction, and severe renal damage if kidney tissue has to be included in the high-dose volume. Surgical excision (colectomy) is the only radical approach. Resection of the involved segment of bowel with a wide margin and its regional lymphatics and nodes, with end-to-end anastomosis, is indicated for lesions above the rectum. Tumours of the rectum require abdominoperineal resection.

Cytotoxic chemotherapy has a place in the palliative management of colonic adenocarcinoma; fluorouracil as a single agent will produce a response in about 10% of cases.

Rectal adenocarcinomas are less radioresistant, and marked regression can be achieved at dose levels which permit subsequent surgical excision. Combined radiotherapy and surgery has its advocates, therefore. After radiotherapy alone, even at high doses, recurrence is frequent.

Palliative radiotherapy is of some value for the relief of pain from pelvic or perineal tumour masses. Responses to cytotoxic chemotherapy are poor.

Results

Reported results for early localised tumours of the large bowel are about 80% at 5 years overall, for tumours with proximal lymph node involvement about 40%, and for tumours with more distant node involvement about 20%.

Anal canal and anus

The mucosal lining of the anal canal differs from that of the rectum, being of cutaneous type. Therefore, the majority of cancers in this area are squamous cell carcinomas. The anus itself is covered by normal skin, and occasionally basal cell carcinomas are seen. Malignant melanomas occasionally arise in either area. Females are affected a little more frequently than males. Leukoplakia may undergo malignant change, and it has been suggested that haemorrhoids and fistulae predispose to carcinoma.

Most tumours are ulcerated and infiltrating. Lymphatic drainage is to the groin nodes, but deposits from extensive tumours may be found in the iliac and para-aortic nodes.

Symptoms

Early symptoms are local irritation and discomfort; later, tenesmus, discharge and bleeding may be features. Pain is a late symptom.

Treatment

Early lesions of the anus can be excised without damaging the sphincter muscles; more extensive lesions and those of the anal canal require sacrifice of the sphincters at abdominoperineal resection.

In selected cases, radiotherapy may be effective with preservation of sphincter function. A localised anal carcinoma can be implanted with radiocaesium needles, but normal tissue tolerance in this area is limited. Preliminary colostomy has much to offer by directing the bowel contents away from the tumour area during the phase of radiation reaction and tumour regression. Often, the bowel continuity can be restored when healing is complete.

External beam-directed high-energy radiation therapy may be of some value in the palliation of advanced tumours; the alternative of colostomy alone may be equally effective and less upsetting. Bleomycin has also been reported to be of some value.

Operable inguinal lymph node deposits are treated by block dissection of the groin.

Results

Five-year survival figures of about 65% are quoted for early lesions. The corresponding figure for more advanced but operable tumours is about 50%.

Chapter 9
Head and Neck Cancer

The head and neck region contains a multitude of tissues and structures from which a wide variety of malignant tumours arise. For detailed consideration the region can be subdivided conveniently into areas and organs, thus:

1 Lip.
2 Mouth,
   a tongue,
   b floor of mouth,
   c buccal and gingival mucosa,
   d mandible and maxilla,
   e palate.
3 Tonsillar area and oropharynx.
4 Postnasal space.
5 Nasal cavity and paranasal sinuses.
6 Larynx and hypopharynx,
   a larynx,
   b hypopharynx.
7 Eye and orbit,
   a eyelids,
   b eye,
   c orbital cavity.
8 Salivary glands.
9 Thyroid and parathyroids.
10 Middle ear cleft.

Lymphatic drainage

An essential part of the management of some malignant tumours in the head and neck area is the treatment of regional lymph node metastases. About 90% of such tumours of the lips and buccal cavity are squamous carcinomas, which metastasise mainly via the lymphatics. Therefore, a review of the local lymphatic system is appropriate.

The lymph nodes draining the region are concentrated mainly in the preauricular, submental, submandibular and deep cervical areas. The deep

97

cervical chain is divided into upper, middle and lower groups for descriptive purposes.

The lymphatic drainage of the lips is to the submental, submandibular and upper deep cervical nodes. The middle third of the lower lip drains to the submental group; the outer parts of the lower lip and the upper lip drain to the submandibular group. There may be some drainage directly to the upper deep cervical group, and rarely also to the pre-auricular area.

The lymphatics from the anterior two-thirds of the tongue drain mainly to the middle deep cervical group; the tip also drains to the submental nodes and the lateral borders to the submandibular nodes. The posterior third drains to the upper deep cervical nodes and vessels may cross the midline. Drainage from the floor of the mouth is similar to that from the lateral border of the tongue, but again bilateral flow is not uncommon.

The buccal mucosa and alveolar areas drain to the submandibular and upper deep cervical nodes; so do the palatal lymphatics.

Lymphatics from the tonsillar area and the oropharynx pass to the upper deep cervical nodes. The postnasal space lymphatics drain to the same nodes and also to the retropharyngeal nodes, commonly to both sides of the midline. Drainage of the nasal cavity and paranasal sinuses is by similar routes, commonly bilaterally from the nasal cavity but not from the major sinuses. The lymphatics from the orbit and from the middle ear cleft drain mainly to the upper deep cervical nodes.

The laryngeal lymphatics and those from the postcricoid region pass to the lower deep cervical group and to paratracheal and retrosternal nodes. Somewhat surprisingly, those from the pyriform fossa pass to the upper deep cervical nodes. Again, bilateral drainage is common.

Drainage from the thyroid gland is to the deep cervical chain, the level depending upon the level in the organ from which the vessels originate.

It should be noted that the commonest primary carcinomas producing neck node metastases in males of middle and old age arise in the head and neck region.

The only potentially curative treatment for lymph node metastases from epithelial tumours in the head and neck region is radical block dissection. This operation entails the meticulous *en bloc* removal of the sternomastoid muscle, internal jugular vein, upper middle and lower deep cervical, submandibular and submental lymph nodes and submandibular salivary gland, and the nodes in the supraclavicular fossa and posterior triangle of neck, with all the intervening lymphatic channels and connective tisue. The resulting disfiguration is surprisingly little.

Tumour involvement beyond lymph node capsules contraindicates the operation; attempted removal usually results in wider dissemination of tumour foci in the tissues.

Bilateral block dissections can be performed, but not simultaneously, and if possible with the preservation of the internal jugular vein on one side.

Lip

The commonest site of malignant tumours in the mouth area, accounting for about 25%. Tumours of the lower lip are about ten times commoner than upper lip tumours. They are predominantly tumours of later life.

Malignant tumours of the lip are similar to those of the skin elsewhere and of the buccal cavity, but carcinomas tend to produce lymph node metastases earlier. Being clearly visible, they usually present early, and most carcinomas can be cured by radiotherapy, with good functional and cosmetic results.

The classical tumour is the squamous cell carcinoma, usually well differentiated. It can present as an ulcer with indurated base, a plaque, a fissure, or an exophytic growth. Much less frequently basal cell carcinomas arise, and occasionally malignant melanomas are seen. Rarely, malignant salivary tissue tumours arise in the substance of the lip. Biopsy confirmation is mandatory and is usually easily obtained.

Predisposing factors include leucoplakia and prolonged exposure to sunlight.

Management

Management depends upon the site and histological nature of the lesion. Carcinomas, if not too extensive, are amenable to irradiation or surgical excision. Radiation therapy does not involve further tissue loss and produces a better functional and cosmetic result, and is to be preferred in most cases. Surgery is available for residual or recurrent disease. Malignant salivary gland tumours and melanomas should be excised if possible.

Unilateral regional lymph node deposits are treated by radical block dissection, if this is technically possible. Operable nodes in patients unfit for operation can be irradiated, but the chances of success are less than from block dissection. Inoperable deposits may show some response with useful growth restraint from radiotherapy.

Results

Early carcinomas of the lip treated by irradiation or surgery yield 5-year survival figures of about 90%; the incidence of recurrent disease beyond this interval is minimal.

Mouth

Tongue

The tongue is the second commonest site of malignant tumours in the mouth area (about 20%). Again, males are affected much more often than females, and the disease is predominantly one of later life.

Aetiological factors include chronic irritation, as from a sharp tooth, habitual tongue biting, and leucoplakia.

The tongue can be divided into the anterior two-thirds and the posterior third in respect of tumour type and differentiation, lymphatic spread and natural history. About three-quarters of tumours arise on the anterior two-thirds, the commonest sites being the lateral border, dorsum, tip and under surface, in decreasing order of frequency. Macroscopically lesions may be solid and nodular, softer and papillary, flat and plaque-like, ulcerated and indurated, or fissured. Histologically, almost all are squamous carcinomas, and mainly of well-differentiated type. Adenocarcinomas occasionally arise from mucous glands of salivary tissue. Melanomas rarely occur.

Tumours of the posterior third of the tongue tend to be less differentiated; lymphomas, predominantly of non-Hodgkin's type, are occasionally seen.

Symptoms

The symptoms of early disease are none or minimal. Local pain and ulceration may develop late. Reduced mobility of the tongue with dysphagia is usually also a late feature. There may be excessive salivation. Posterior third lesions may present as persistent 'sore throat'. At presentation lymph node involvement is evident in about one-third of anterior lesions and in about two-thirds of posterior lesions.

Treatment

The classical form of treatment for a carcinoma of the middle third of the lateral border is the single plane interstitial needle implant. This has been so for many decades, and still is true; the only difference being that radiocaesium needles are now usually used instead of the traditional radium ones. Surgery is an alternative, and is equally effective, but inevitably results in tissue loss and reduced functional efficiency. More advanced lesions of the anterior parts and most lesions of the posterior part require radiotherapy.

Involved neck nodes are managed as for those from carcinoma of the lip.

Results

Quoted results are an overall 5-year survival of about 30%—about 70% for early lesions of the anterior two-thirds, and less for posterior third lesions.

Vallecula and epiglottis

Tumours of the vallecula and anterior surface of the epiglottis can be considered in this section. Most malignant tumours are squamous cell carcinomas. Dysphagia is the usual presenting symptom. Bilateral lymph node involvement is not uncommon. Surgery has little to offer and full-dose radiotherapy is the only hope of eradicating these tumours.

Floor of mouth

The floor of the mouth accounts for some 15% of malignant mouth tumours. Again they are commoner in males than in females. Heavy smoking and drinking and ill-fitting dentures are suggested predisposing factors. Almost all are squamous carcinomas. Local extension to the mandible and root of the tongue occurs early, and these tumours often cross the midline.

Management

Management is usually by irradiation of the primary tumour; treatment of the neck noded deposits follows the same lines as for lip lesions.

Results

Results quoted for tumours without node involvement are up to 70% at 5 years; this figure is halved if the neck nodes are involved.

Buccal and gingival mucosa

These sites account for another 15% or so of mouth tumours, and yet again are commoner in males than in females. The classical association between buccal mucosa carcinoma and the sucking of a plug made from betel nut, tobacco and slaked lime, kept in the sulcus, is often quoted, but is relevant mainly to natives of South-East Asia, southern India and the Philipines, and therefore in Britain is of limited importance.

Leucoplakia is a common predisposing condition. Almost all tumours are squamous carcinomas; a few malignant tumours of salivary tissue and melanomas are reported.

Local infiltration into the pterygoid fossa produces trismus, but usually this is a late feature. Earlier symptoms are related to local ulceration.

Treatment

Surgery to the primary tumour, to be effective, must be extensive and mutilating. Nevertheless, it is the treatment of choice if there is local bone involvement, as radiotherapy is then less effective. Otherwise, radiotherapy is to be preferred. For lymph node deposits the only potentially curative treatment is radical block dissection of the neck.

Results

Quoted figures for the treatment of early tumours are about 70% survival at 5 years; local lymph node involvement reduces this figure to about half (35%).

Mandible and maxilla

Malignant tumours in these bones include fibrosarcoma and osteosarcoma (rarely). Another tumour of interest is the adamantinoma, also known as ameloblastoma. It is rare except in parts of Africa. It affects females more often than males, is commoner in the mandible than the maxilla, and has its highest incidence in the age range 20-40 years. It arises from epithelial remnants in the bone, with solid tumour areas and cystic fluid-filled spaces. Rarely, malignant forms are described.

Treatment

Treatment of all these tumours is surgical excision if technically possible; radiotherapy can be of only palliative value.

Benign conditions which can be confused include Paget's disease, fibrous dysplasia, aneurysmal bone cyst, the lipoid storage diseases, and giant cell midline granuloma. Biopsy confirmation of the diagnosis is therefore mandatory.

Results

Results of treatment depend upon the tumour type. Quoted figures for fibrosarcoma and osteosarcoma are similar to those for tumours in other bones (see Chapter 14); adamantinomas yield cure rates of about 80%.

Palate

Tumours in this area are uncommon. On the hard palate, tumours of salivary tissue predominate; they arise in younger subjects than most other mouth tumours, and one variety is cylindroma. This tumour extends slowly but remorselessly, with microscopic extent well beyond that apparent clinically, and it has a marked tendency to produce lung metastases. Tumours of the soft palate are mainly of squamous type. Neck node involvement occurs fairly early.

Surgical excision is indicated for tumours of salivary tissue, with provision of a prosthesis to occlude the defect produced. Radiotherapy is indicated for squamous carcinomas.

Results

Results quoted are 5-year survival rates of about 60% for early lesions, and about 30% for more advanced lesions.

Tonsillar area and oropharynx

The majority of malignant tumours in these areas arise from the mucosa and not from the local lymphoid tissue. These carcinomas are usually poorly differentiated, and present as exophytic and ulcerated lesions. They affect males about nine times more frequently than females.

In the tonsillar area extension soon leads to involvement of the faucial pillars, soft palate, retromolar fossa, base of tongue and lateral wall of the pharynx. Deep extension produces trismus. Lymphatic spread occurs early.

Tumours may arise primarily in the pharyngeal mucosa; those on the posterior wall tend to extend slowly and to metastasise late because of the dense prevertebral fascia and the relative sparcity of lymphatics in the area.

Management

Management of carcinomas is essentially by radiotherapy. Malignant lymphoma of the tonsil is more commonly of non-Hodgkin than of Hodgkin type, and management is the same as that for lymphomas elsewhere. Carcinomas arising on the soft palate and uvula are rare. They are said to be more resistant to radiotherapy than lesions in the faucial region.

Results

Results achieved for early carcinomas without lymph node involvement are about 45% at 5 years; neck node involvement reduces this to about

20%. Results of treatment of lymphomas are about 45% at 5 years overall, with significantly better figures for early stage disease.

Postnasal space

This is a small cavity, but malignant tumours arising from its walls can have marked effects, as a result of local infiltration and lymphatic spread.

In most parts of the world, the incidence is low (about 1% of all malignancies), but in China and South-East Asia it is much higher. It has been suggested that the latter is associated with infection with the Epstein–Barr virus.

The commonest malignant tumour is the squamous cell carcinoma, usually poorly differentiated, and sometimes showing lymphocytic infiltration (lymphoepithelioma). Transitional cell carcinomas are described, and occasionally lymphomas arise in this area. Chordoma, a tumour of notocord remnants, may present in the postnasal space. Plasmacytomas and tumours of salivary gland tissue are also described.

Increasing local tumour bulk may cause nasal obstruction, discharge and bleeding, and occlusion of the Eustachian tube with deafness. The soft palate may be displaced downwards. Infiltration in the lateral and posterior walls is directed upwards by the dense pharyngeal fascia, with invasion of the foraminae in the base of the skull and involvement of the bone itself; cranial nerve palsies result—3rd, 4th, 5th and 6th, at the foramen lacerum, and 9th, 10th, 11th and 12th, in the region of the foramen ovale. The tumour may extend into the orbit and produce proptosis.

Lymph node deposits develop early, and both sides of the neck may be affected. Indeed, the primary tumour may be small and asymptomatic, and the neck node involvement may draw attention to the condition. Node involvement may extend to the supraclavicular fossa and the upper mediastinum.

Investigations

Radiology is of great value in diagnosis and assessment. Base of skull views will indicate any bone destruction, and contrast studies with radio-opaque fluid in the postnasal space will clearly define the extent of the soft-tissue mass. CT scanning may also be of great value.

Treatment

Treatment is by irradiation. For poorly differentiated carcinomas the volume to be covered must be great, extending from above the base of the skull to the mediastinum.

Results

Overall 5-year survival figures of about 30% are quoted; for early tumours the figure is about 60%.

Nasal cavity and paranasal sinuses

These must be considered as a whole, as the intercommunications between the nasal cavity and the sinuses often lead to extensive involvement of both by malignant tumours.

Tumour types include squamous cell carcinoma (about 80%), malignant salivary tumours, malignant melanoma, lymphoma and fibrosarcoma. The incidence is higher in males than in females, and woodworkers (especially cabinet makers) show an increased incidence due to inhaled wood dust. There may be a long history of chronic nasal catarrh and polyposis.

The commonest site of origin is the maxillary sinus (antrum). It is a small cavity, and symptoms and signs are usually related to extension through the antral walls. Medial extension produces nasal obstruction, discharge and bleeding. Extension anteriorly leads to swelling of the cheek, initially in the malar area, and often with local pain and discomfort. Posterior extension into the pterygoid fossa produces trismus. Upward extension through the thin bony floor of the orbit leads to diplopia and proptosis, and may result in numbness of the cheek due to involvement of the maxillary division of the trigeminal nerve. Extension downwards produces swelling of the palate, alveolus or bucco-alveolar sulcus, and antral tumours may present initially in this area.

In the nasal cavity common sites of origin are the septum and the turbinates (especially the inferior which is the largest). The ethmoid air cells are seldom involved alone, but are often affected in association with antral tumours. The classical sign is swelling in the inner canthus of the eye. Frontal sinus tumours are very uncommon, and sphenoidal sinus tumours are rare.

Clinical examination will give a good indication of the site of origin and extent of these tumours, but radiology is of great value in defining accurately the tumour limits, CT scanning being especially helpful. Biopsy is essential; for antral tumours this is obtained by the Cauldwell–Luc approach through the canine fossa, which also establishes drainage.

Treatment

Treatment is by irradiation after drainage has been obtained, either as above, or by a hemipalatectomy. Often, the antrum, nasal cavity (both sides), ethmoid cells and orbit must be treated in one block. Inevitably this means including the eye in the high-dose volume, with resultant cataract formation, since attempts to shield the eye may leave tumour not treated to adequate dose.

After radiotherapy, some authorities advocate hemipalatectomy (if not done initially) to ensure continued drainage of the cavity and to allow easier inspection at follow-up.

Results

Overall results show about a 30% 5-year survival.

Larynx and hypopharynx

Larynx

Malignant tumours of the larynx account for about one-fifth of all head and neck cancers. Males are affected nine times more frequently than females, and almost all tumours are squamous cell carcinomas. The most definite aetiological factor is smoking; industrial atmospheric polution has also been incriminated.

The intrinsic larynx can be divided into three areas:

1 Supraglottic area—from the tip of the epiglottis, free edge of the aryepiglottic fold and upper surface of the arytenoids, down to the laryngeal ventricle.

2 Glottic area—the true cords and the anterior commissure.

3 Subglottic area—from the undersurface of the true cords downwards for an arbitrary 1 cm.

The majority of laryngeal carcinomas arise in the glottic area, on the true cord, usually starting in the anterior third and spreading directly to the anterior commissure and opposite cord, to the arytenoid region and to the ventricle and subglottic area. Lateral extension results in reduced mobility of the cord.

These are few lymphatic vessels in the true cord, and lymph node deposits from early tumours are uncommon. However, once a tumour has spread beyond the cord it reaches tissue profusely supplied with lymphatics and node deposits are common. Supraglottic and subglottic tumours tend to produce lymph node deposits much earlier in their course.

Symptoms

Hoarseness is the only early symptom of glottic carcinoma, and hoarseness persisting for more than 4 weeks should be regarded with suspicion. It may be intermittent initially but later becomes continuous. Later symptoms include local pain and dysphagia, irritant cough and dyspnoea.

Investigations

Indirect and direct laryngoscopy are helpful in diagnosis and assessment; the former allows cord movement to be checked and the latter allows a biopsy to be taken. Tomograms are also useful, especially in assessing extension to the ventricle and subglottic area.

Treatment

Radiotherapy for early laryngeal carcinoma offers excellent prospects of cure and of restoring a voice of good quality.

Laryngectomy may be effective for residual or recurrent disease.

More extensive tumours with cord fixation or subglottic spread are better treated by laryngectomy. Palliative radiotherapy may be indicated for advanced tumours with inoperable neck node metastases. Preliminary tracheostomy may be necessary.

Tumours arising in the supraglottic and subglottic areas are treated surgically in most centres, but radical radiotherapy has a place in the management of supraglottic lesions.

Results

Early tumours yield 5-year survival figures of about 85%; for more advanced tumours the figure falls to about 30%.

Hypopharnyx

The two sites in the hypopharynx from which malignant tumours most commonly arise are the pyriform fossa and the postcricoid area.

Pyriform fossa

Tumours of the pyriform fossa are much commoner in males than females (9 : 1). This may be related in part to smoking and drinking habits (alcohol). Squamous cell carcinoma is the common lesion; other rarer tumours include adenocarcinoma and melanoma.

Lymph node metastases develop early, and may be evident before there are any symptoms referrable to the primary tumour.

Medial spread of the tumour produces discomfort in the throat, dysphagia and hoarseness; lateral extension may make the primary mass palpable externally. Pain referred to the ear is not uncommon. The upper part of the tumour may be visible on indirect examination; direct examination will be more informative. Radiological lateral soft-tissue views of the neck and tomograms of the laryngeal area are helpful.

Many authorities advocate radical surgery in the form of laryngopharyngectomy; other claim that localised disease can be eradicated by full-dose radiotherapy, which preserves the normal swallowing pathway.

Results of treatment are not good; early lesions without node involvement yield 5-year survival figures of about 35%.

Postcricoid area

Tumours of the postcricoid area are much commoner in females than in males (again 9 : 1). They arise classically in small, thin, frail women, with smooth skin, fissures at the corners of the mouth, spoon-shaped nails, an oesophageal web, atrophic mucosa in the upper alimentary tract and stomach, achlorhydria and iron-deficiency anaemia (Plummer–Vinson or Paterson–Brown–Kelly syndrome).

Dysphagia is the main symptom. Later there may be overspill of fluids and food into the larynx with fits of coughing. Lymph node deposits occur early.

Direct examination will reveal the tumour, which may be exophytic or infiltrating and stenosing, and will allow a biopsy to be taken. Often there is pooled mucus and saliva behind the larynx. Cautious barium swallow is helpful in assessing the length of the lesion.

Radical radiotherapy may be effective for early tumours. If the lesion has encircled the pharynx, healing may result in a fibrous stricture, which may require regular dilatation. However, successful radiotherapy again maintains the natural pathway for swallowing. Radical surgical treatment is by laryngopharyngectomy.

Yet again, results are not good, with overall 5-year survival rates of about 25% being reported.

Eye and orbit

Treatment of malignant tumours of the eye and orbit aims at eradication of the disease, and if possible preservation of sight; the former, of course, must take precedence.

The lens of the eye is very sensitive to radiation damage; the cornea itself is more resistant, but is sensitive to changes in the conjunctiva and uveal tract. The retina is even more resistant, and the sclera shows little evidence of damage at full doses.

Eyelids

Tumours include basal and squamous cell carcinomas, malignant melanoma, and adenocarcinoma of the Meibomian glands.

Carcinomas are treated by irradiation, using a lead shield to protect the eye; superficial radiation is usually adequate. Melanomas and adenocarcinomas are excised.

Eye

The commonest tumours are retinoblastoma and malignant melanoma. Retinoblastoma is considered in Chapter 12.

Malignant melanoma of the eye is rare. It may be circumscribed or diffuse. Local extension occurs early; metastases, classically to the liver but also to the brain, arise early but may not become evident for many years.

These tumours occur mainly in adults, who complain of visual disturbance or of pain in the eye as the presenting symptom.

They are radioresistant and excision is the only effective treatment, although local recurrence or residue after surgery may be controlled by radiotherapy to full dose.

Overall 5-year survival figures of about 50% have been repoted.

Metastases in the eye occasionally arise, the commonest primary sites being the breast and bronchus.

Orbital cavity

Primary malignant tumours, excluding those of the eye itself, include lacrymal gland tumours (adenocarcinoma and lymphoma), sarcomas (rhabdomyosarcoma and fibrosarcoma), and optic nerve tumours (glioma and meningioma). Metastases occur occasionally, the classical primary being neuroblastoma.

Tumours in the orbital cavity produce diplopia, displacement of the eye and proptosis, but no impairment of vision occurs until a late stage.

Lacrymal gland tumours are excised if possible; radiotherapy is of limited value but may be useful as palliation. Rhabdomyosarcoma may respond well to combined surgery, radiotherapy and cytotoxic chemotherapy. Fibrosarcoma is radioresistant, and surgery is the only available form of radical treatment. Meningioma is also radioresistant, but gliomas may show a limited response if poorly differentiated.

Useful palliation may be achieved from irradiation of metastases; neuroblastoma deposits being particularly sensitive.

Salivary gland tumours

Tumours of salivary tissue may arise in the major glands (parotid, submandibular and sublingual) or in the numerous small collections of tissue in the walls of the upper alimentary tract. The parotid gland is by far the commonest site.

About one-third of tumours are malignant, with highest incidence above the age of 60 years. Benign tumours are more common 10–20 years earlier.

Commoner tumours may be classified as in Table 9.1.

Table 9.1. Classification of salivary tumours.

BENIGN

1 Mixed salivary tumour (pleomorphic adenoma), showing epithelial and cartilage-like cells and fibrous tissue with mucin present
2 Adenolymphoma, an adenoma with lymphocytic infiltration

MALIGNANT

1 Malignant mixed tumours, showing cytological evidence of malignancy and invasion of the capsule
2 Adenocarcinoma, arising in the secreting alveoli
3 Cylindroma, a form of adenocarcinoma which shows a typical cylindrical arrangement of cells, and infiltrates widely
4 Mucoepidermoid carcinoma, arising from duct epithelium
5 Lymphoma

Mixed salivary tumours

Mixed salivary tumours are commonest in the major glands, and particularly in the parotid. They are not very radiosensitive, and excision is the treatment of choice. However, complete removal of parotid adenomas is difficult because of their close relation to the branches of the facial nerve. Adenomas in this and other glands are also difficult to remove fully because although they appear macroscopically to have a well-defined capsule, buds of tumour extend beyond this. Tumours of the submandibular and sublingual glands can be excised with the whole gland.

Recurrence of mixed salivary tumours is therefore not uncommon, and full-dose radiotherapy may be indicated.

Malignant salivary tumours

Malignant salivary tumours are also not very radiosensitive, and again excision is the treatment of choice, with sacrifice of the branches of the facial nerve for parotid tumours if complete clearance is thereby possible. If there is residual tumour after surgery, or excision is not possible, radiotherapy is needed.

Five-year survival figures for malignant tumours are quoted as about 50%.

Thyroid

Malignant tumours of the thyroid are rare; on average there are twelve new cases for every one million of the population each year, although they are said to be commoner in goitrous areas of the world (e.g. Derbyshire and Switzerland). They are commoner in females than in males in the ratio 2 : 1. There is statistical evidence to suggest that Hashimoto's disease is a predisposing factor.

Malignant thyroid tumours can be classified as follows:

1 Well-differentiated carcinomas,
  a mainly papillary,
  b mainly follicular.
2 Anaplastic carcinoma.
3 Medullary carcinoma.
4 Lymphoma.

Well-differentiated tumours occur in the age range 10–50 years. They may retain some functional ability, and therefore may take up radioiodine. Anaplastic tumours occur in an older age group (60–80 years), and have no hormonal function. Medullary carcinoma is not strictly a thyroid tumour, arising from the C cells of the gland, and may excrete excess of calcitonin (see Chapter 16). Lymphoma is usually of non-Hodgkin's type. Papillary carcinomas spread mainly via the lymphatics; follicular carcinomas mainly via the bloodstream. Anaplastic carcinomas are locally invasive and may metastasise widely to lymph nodes and other organs.

Investigations

Investigations include thyroid function tests, thyroid antibody titres, radiographs (of chest, thoracic inlet and the skeleton), and radioisotope uptake measurements and scans of the neck and other areas of the body as indicated.

Management

External radiotherapy has no place in the management of well-differentiated carcinomas. For papillary tumours, total thyroidectomy or partial resection (of one lobe and the isthmus) with block dissection of the neck on the side of the major thyroid involvement, is indicated. After partial thyroidectomy thyroid hormone suppression therapy is given. After total thyroidectomy with demonstrable residue or metastases on scans, an ablation dose of radioiodine-131 is given, with repeat scans every 3–6 months and further doses of the isotope if any functioning tissue is detected. Further surgery may be indicated for local residue in the neck.

For follicular tumours, total thyroidectomy is needed followed by scanning and an ablation dose of radioiodine. Thyroid hormone suppression then is started. Repeat scans and radioiodine therapy may be required as for papillary tumours.

Surgery in the management of anaplastic thyroid carcinoma is limited to biopsy, or to removal of the main bulk of the tumour and to the relief of pressure symptoms. Thereafter, thyroid hormone replacement is started, and palliative radiotherapy given to the primary area, upper mediastinum, neck and supraclavicular lymph node areas. Cytotoxic chemotherapy has no defined place in management.

Medullary carcinoma is treated by total thyroidectomy with block dissection of the neck if indicated, followed by thyroid hormone replacement.

Lymphoma of the thyroid is treated by irradiation (similar to that given for lymphoma arising in the neck glands) after surgery as for anaplastic carcinoma, and with thyroid hormone replacement as necessary.

Results

Five-year survival figures of 80–90% are claimed for the treatment of early papillary carcinomas, and 50–60% for follicular carcinomas. These figures fall to about 30% if metastases are present. Survival for anaplastic carcinomas is worse, with figures of about 10% at 5 years. The overall survival of lymphoma of the gland is about 45% at 5 years.

Hyperthyroidism

Hyperthyroidism is not a malignant condition, but radioiodine has an established place in its management. Alternative forms of treatment are antithyroid drugs and subtotal thyroidectomy, both of which have significant side effects or dangers, for example blood dyscrasias from the drugs and recurrent laryngeal nerve palsy, tetany and hypothyroidism from surgery.

Radioiodine therapy is simple and safe, and has no side effects except for a gradually rising incidence of hypothyroidism with the passage of time after treatment, and possible genetic effects. The former calls for long-term follow-up of treated patients, and the latter dictates that treatment is confined in women to those over the age of 40 years.

No statistically significant increase in the incidence of leukaemia or thyroid malignancy after radioiodine therapy for thyrotoxicosis has been reported.

Parathyroid tumours

Parathyroid tumours produce excess of parathormone, and the resulting features are primarily due to disturbances in calcium and phosphorus handling by the gut, bone and kidneys. Hypercalcaemia is seen in association with the classical bone disease of osteitis fibrosa cystica (von Recklinghausen's disease). Most parathyroid tumours are benign, although carcinoma does rarely occur. Treatment is by surgery, and results are usually good.

Middle ear cleft

This includes the middle ear cavity, mastoid air cells, and adjacent petrous bone. Malignant disease in these areas is uncommon. Most malignant tumours are squamous cell carcinomas (80%), and the only other tumour of interest is that of the glomus jugulare.

Squamous cell carcinoma may arise in the skin of the external auditory meatus, in the middle ear cavity or in the mastoid air cells. Chronic middle ear infection is a recognised predisposing factor.

Local extension may be slow, but metastases in the neck glands are present in about 10% of cases at presentation. Symptoms include discharge (often bloodstained), local pain and deafness. Investigations include radiography of the skull with tomograms of the relevant area.

Management

In management, radical surgery to the primary tumour is of limited value, but is indicated for operable neck node deposits, and is helpful in establishing drainage. Control of infection is also important. The mainstay of treatment is radical beam-directed radiotherapy.

Results

Results of treatment are not impressive; 5-year survival figures of about 25% are quoted.

Glomus jugulare tumours

Glomus jugulare tumour or chemodectoma, arises in the petrous-mastoid bone from a structure histologically similar to the carotid body in the neck.

It can present as deafness, watery bloodstained or purulent discharge, tinnitus, pain or vertigo. Granulation tissue or a polyp may be visible deep in the external auditory meatus or behind the tympanic membrane. Cranial nerves may be involved, most commonly the 10th and 12th, but also the 7th, 9th and 11th. Radiographs will show local bone destruction.

Surgery again is of limited value, and may be associated with profuse bleeding. Radiotherapy to fairly high doses can lead to prolonged control of the tumour, with healing or partial healing, cessation of bleeding and discharge, relief of pain, and improvement in nerve palsies in some cases. Response is slow, and may extend over 6 months or more.

Carotid body tumours

Carotid body tumour arises in the structure of that name at the bifurcation of the common carotid artery. It is slow growing, usually presents in the third or fourth decade of life, and rarely shows malignant features such as local invasion or metastases. If treatment is indicated, surgical excision is the only form, and this may be hazardous because of profuse bleeding.

Cytotoxic chemotherapy

Cytotoxic chemotherapy in head and neck cancer may be of value in the management of advanced or recurrent squamous carcinomas not amenable to surgery. Drugs which have shown some responses include vincristine, bleomycin, cyclophosphamide and methotrexate. Usually they are used in combination, but bleomycin has been advocated alone or in conjunction with radiotherapy.

Chapter 10
Cancer of the Genitourinary Tract

This will be considered under the following headings:
1 Female genital tract,
   a uterine cervix,
   b endometrium,
   c ovary,
   d vagina and vulva,
   e choriocarcinoma.
2 Male genital tract,
   a testis,
   b prostate,
   c penis.
3 Urinary tract,
   a kidney, renal pelvis and ureter, and adrenal gland,
   b bladder,
   c urethra.

Female genital tract

Uterine cervix

Cancer of the uterine cervix is the second commonest malignancy in females, accounting for about 12% of cases; the commonest is breast cancer.

Aetiology

The age of first intercourse and of first pregnancy are important factors in aetiology. The epithelium of the cervix undergoes metaplastic changes at puberty and during the early weeks of first pregnancy, and at these times spermatozoa can be incorporated into the tissue with possible carcinogenic effects. Promiscuity, high parity, and low social status are associated with an increased incidence of cervical cancer; the latter is thought to be related in part to vitamin-A deficiency. It has been suggested that a virus (probably herpes simplex or papilloma virus) is also a factor in aetiology.

Circumcision of male partners is well recognised as being associated with a low incidence of the disease. The highest incidence is in the 45-55 age range.

Pathology

About 95% of cancers are squamous cell carcinomas, arising from the epithelium of the vaginal cervix or endocervical canal. About 5% are adenocarcinomas arising from the endocervix. Rarely, mixed mesodermal tumour (sarcoma botryoides) is reported in childhood. Invasive squamous carcinoma may be preceded by *in situ* malignant change for 10 years or more. However, in only about one-third of cases does the *in situ* change progress to frank malignancy. Nevertheless, routine cervical smear examination can detect those at risk, so that treatment or close follow-up can be instituted. Tumours may be exophytic or infiltrating and ulcerative.

Locally the disease spreads to the fornices, the upper vaginal wall and the uterine body. Lymphatic spread is to the broad ligaments and utero-sacral ligaments, and to the external iliac, common iliac and para-aortic nodes. Haematogenous spread is less common, with metastases in the brain, lungs and ovaries. In most cases, however, the disease remains confined to the pelvis until very advanced.

Symptoms

Early cervical carcinomas are asymptomatic, and the diagnosis may be made on routine examination and cervical smear cytology. Later, bleeding and discharge are features; the bleeding may be postcoital, intermenstrual or postmenopausal; the discharge often is bloodstained and offensive. Later still, there may be pain due to lumbosacral nerve involvement. Advanced local disease may produce a vesicovaginal or rectovaginal fistula, or ureteric obstruction.

Investigations

Investigations include full blood count, plasma urea and electrolyte estimations, chest X-ray films, bilateral lower limb lymphograms, and intravenous pyelography. Cystoscopy is essential to determine any bladder base invasion. Biopsy is mandatory.

Clinical staging

Clinical staging is an essential preliminary to determining management. Although a TNM classification and staging is available, many centres still use an older system, one form of which is shown in Table 10.1.

Table 10.1. Clinical staging of cervical carcinoma.

---

0 Carcinoma *in situ*
1 Confined to the cervix
  (a) Microinvasive
  (b) Clinically evident
II (a) Extension to the upper two-thirds of vagina
  (b) Extension to the parametria, but not to the pelvic side wall
III Extension to the lower third of the vagina or to the pelvic side wall
IV Involvement of the bladder or rectum or extension outside the pelvis

---

Staging is done under general anaesthesia so that relaxation is good. At the same time, cystoscopy is performed, a biopsy is taken, and dilatation and curettage are done to detect any involvement of the uterine body or pyometra. It must be emphasised that staging is clinical, taking into account cystoscopic but not lymphographic findings.

Treatment

For all but stage 0 and stage IV cases, treatment is usually a combination of intracavitary radioisotope and high-energy external radiation therapy. The commonly used radioisotope is caesium-137.

The radioisotope is mounted in applicators suitable for insertion into the cervical canal and upper vagina. They are introduced under general anaesthesia.

Stage 0 disease usually is treated surgically. In younger women who desire to have children, cone biopsy may be adequate but may also reduce the chances of pregnancy; in older women simple hysterectomy is the treatment of choice. Diathermy or laser therapy are now accepted treatment in younger women, if there is adequate colposcopic follow-up. If stage 0 disease is detected in pregnancy, the latter can be allowed to go to term, and treatment of the malignancy instituted if necessary thereafter; *in situ* carcinoma of pregnancy can regress spontaneously.

For stage I and stage II disease, one standard technique consists of two radiocaesium insertions 1 week apart initially. For stage III disease, a single insertion is given initially. In all of these stages, the dose is supplemented by external high-energy radiation. If there is lymphographic evidence of para-aortic node involvement, the external therapy fields may be extended to cover this.

Stage IV disease confined to the pelvis is treated by external radiotherapy only. The high dose rate from intracavitary radioisotope therapy can result in very rapid initial tumour regression and fistula formation or enlargement of an existing fistula. The lower dose rate from external therapy may allow normal tissue repair to keep pace with the tumour regression and so obviate fistula formation.

Stage IV disease with spread beyond the pelvis, or recurrent disease within the pelvis, may show some response to combination cytotoxic chemotherapy, for example with vinblastine and bleomycin, but results usually are poor.

Some authorities advocate Wertheim's hysterectomy for early malignancy, with or without preliminary intracavitary radiotherapy, but great expertise is required and results in general are poorer than those from radiotherapy. For adenocarcinoma of the cervix, which is less radiosensitive than squamous carcinoma, and for recurrent localised disease, however, this operation may be indicated. As primary treatment it is best combined with preoperative radiotherapy.

Invasive carcinoma diagnosed during pregnancy may be difficult to manage. If the fetus has reached viability (32 weeks) caesarian section is undertaken, and external radiation therapy is started as soon as the skin sutures have been removed. Intracavitary radioisotope therapy then is given, as by this time involution of the uterus will be almost complete. If the pregnancy is less than 24 weeks, therapeutic abortion is to be recommended with radiotherapy immediately thereafter. In the intervening period, each case must be assessed individually, on the extent of the malignancy, on the age and general condition of the patient, on the size of her present family, and on her desire for the current pregnancy to be successful.

Radical radiotherapy often produces temporary tenesmus and diarrhoea, due to reaction in the rectal mucosa, and frequency and dysuria from bladder base reaction towards the end of the treatment and for a week or two thereafter. Late radiation changes can develop in the rectum, bladder and bowel locally, with stricture of the rectum or sigmoid colon and telangiectasia of the bladder base. The latter can be responsible for episodes of haematuria.

Results

Results of treatment, expressed as 5-year survivals, are approximately:
    Stage I—80%
    Stage II—59%
    Stage III—31%
    Stage IV—8%
Overall, about 56% are well at 5 years.

Endometrium

Cancer of the endometrium was less common than that of the uterine cervix, in the raio 1 : 2 or less, but over recent years there has been a gradual tendency for this difference to decrease. It occurs in older women, most arising after the menopause. In contrast to cervical carcinoma it is commoner in the nulliparous and those of low parity. It is said to affect particularly elderly, obese, hypertensive diabetics; in such cases the underlying common factor may be a defect of pituitary function. Endometrial carcinoma may be related to prolonged oestrogen stimulation, either exogenous (e.g. in the treatment of advanced breast cancer or of Turner's syndrome) or endogenous (e.g. from granulosa cell or theca cell tumour of the ovary).

Most cancers are adenocarcinomas, some of which show areas of squamous metaplasia. Rarely, leiomyosarcomas and mixed mesodermal tumours are reported. Endometrial hyperplasia and endometrial polyps are said to be precancerous.

Adenocarcinoma tends to remain localised within the pelvis until a late stage. Invasion of the myometrium is usually slow; spread to the cervix occurs, and deposits in the ovaries, and in the vaginal walls classically just above the urethral meatus, are not uncommon. Lymph node deposits in the iliac and para-aortic areas arise late; blood borne metastases are very uncommon.

Symptoms and diagnosis

The typical symptom of endometrial carcinoma is postmenopausal bleeding, which may be heavy with clots present. In premenopausal women irregular or intermenstrual bleeding is seen. Vaginal discharge is a less common feature. There may be a sense of discomfort in the pelvis. The diagnosis rests on histological examination of uterine curettings. Other investigations include intravenous pyelography, bilateral lower limb lymphography and chest radiography, and assessment of renal function.

Treatment

The best results of treatment for early adenocarcinomas are achieved from a combination of a single intracavitary radiocaesium insertion, and total hysterectomy and bilateral salpingo-oophorectomy either immediately or 6 weeks later. The radiocaesium therapy reduces the incidence of vaginal vault recurrence. If operation reveals extensive myometrial involvement external radiation therapy to the pelvis is given.

In patients unfit for surgery, two radiocaesium insertions 1 week apart may result in good quality and prolonged palliation, but radical intracavitary radiotherapy alone seldom eradicates these tumours.

Local recurrence may respond to external radiotherapy. Distant metastases may show some response to progestogen therapy, for example medroxyprogesterone by mouth, or hydroxyprogesterone hexanoate by intramuscular injection, in high dosage.

Leiomyosarcomas and mixed mesodermal tumours are radioresistant, and the only treatment available is hysterectomy.

Results

Adenocarcinomas confined to the endometrium show 5-year survival rates of about 80%; for more advanced tumours still confined to the uterus figures of about 40% are quoted.

Ovary

Primary malignant tumours of the ovary account for about 20% of those arising in the female genital tract. They may be classified as in Table 10.2.

Epithelial tumours. Cystadenomas represent about 40% of all ovarian tumours. Both serous and mucinous types have a tendency to undergo malignant change, particularly the serous type. They frequently have a papillary structure, the malignant varieties often showing this outside the cyst wall, and seeding throughout the peritoneal cavity.

Cancer has been described as arising in an area of endometriosis (endometrial stromal sarcoma), but usually this is a variety of endometrial

Table 10.2. Classification of ovarian tumours.

EPITHELIAL TUMOURS
Serous cystadenoma and cystadenocarcinoma
Mucinous cystadenoma and cystadenocarcinoma
Endometrial stromal sarcoma
Clear cell (mesonephroid) carcinoma
Brenner tumour
Mixed epithelial tumours
Undifferentiated carcinomas

SEX CORD STROMAL TUMOURS
Granulosa cell tumour, theca cell tumour and fibroma
Arrhenoblastoma

GERM CELL TUMOURS
Dysgerminoma
Teratoma (benign dermoid or malignant teratoma)

CONNECTIVE TISSUE TUMOURS

carcinoma; it may show foci of keratinisation (adenoacanthoma). Clear cell (mesonephroid) carcinoma is probably an undifferentiated epithelial tumour. Brenner tumours almost always are benign and may be very slow growing. Epithelial tumours sometimes contain more than one cell type. The group of undifferentiated carcinomas may represent dysgerminomas, arrhenoblastomas and granulosa cell tumours which show no features to enable more precise identification.

Sex cord stromal tumours. Some ovarian tumours are hormonally active, the commonest being granulosa cell tumours (usually oestrogen secreting) and arrhenoblastomas (usually androgen secreting). Granulosa cell and theca cell elements are present together in some tumours.

Germ cell tumours. Dysgerminoma is the counterpart of the seminoma of testis, and is similarily very radiosensitive. Benign teratoma (dermoid) is relatively common in older women; malignant teratoma of the ovary is rare.

Connective tissue tumours. Fibroma of the ovary is fairly common; fibrosarcoma is rare. Meig's syndrome is an ovarian fibroma with associated ascites and pleural effusions.

In malignant ovarian tumours, in addition to local extension and peritoneal seeding, lymphatic spread to the para-aortic, mediastinal and supraclavicular nodes occurs, and haematogenous dissemination results in lung and liver metastases.

Symptoms and signs

Symptoms and signs may be absent until the disease is locally advanced. The commonest presentation is abdominal swelling due to solid or cystic tumour, ascites, or both. Urinary frequency or incontinence, and diarrhoea or constipation result from local pressure effects. Vague backache is not uncommon, but pain is seldom a feature. Lower limb oedema may develop. Abnormal vaginal bleeding occurs, especially with oestrogen secreting tumours.

Accurate diagnosis rests upon tissue biopsy.

Treatment

Treatment of early tumours is surgical excision. However, many tumours are too advanced. Those still confined to the pelvis may show good palliation from radiotherapy. Cytotoxic chemotherapy may be added with benefit. Thiotepa, cyclophosphamide and cisplatin have been used for the treatment of metastatic disease.

Results

Five-year survival figures of about 60% have been reported for early tumours; once the tumour capsule has been breached the prognosis is much worse, with figures of 10–30%.

Secondary carcinoma

Secondary adenocarcinomas in the ovaries by trans-coelomic spread, Krukenberg tumours, are not uncommon; primary sites include the gastro-intestinal tract (especially the stomach), breast, pancreas and gall bladder.

Vagina

Primary cancer of the vagina is very uncommon; secondary involvement is more common, for example from cervix, endometrium, ovary, kidney or bladder lesions. Most primary carcinomas are of squamous cell type, often due to prolonged use of ring pessaries; a few arise spontaneously. They are commonest in later life. A few arise in childhood, and these can be related to oestrogen therapy to the mother during pregnancy and lactation.

The tumour may be of proliferative or of infiltrating ulcerative type. Spread occurs locally, and via the lymphatics to the pelvic and para-aortic nodes from upper vaginal lesions and to the groin nodes from lower lesions.

Symptoms

Bleeding is the usual presenting symptom.

Treatment

Upper and middle third lesions are treated as for carcinoma of the cervix; localised lower third lesions may be implantable with radioactive needles, with external radiation therapy to the pelvic lymph nodes if involved.

Vulva

Cancer of the vulva is also uncommon. Again, most carcinomas are of squamous cell type, and again are commonest in later life. They may be associated with chronic irritative conditions of the vulval skin which may be related to poor hygiene. Venereal granulomas, leukoplakia and vulval warts occasionally undergo malignant change.

Lymphatic spread is to the inguinal nodes initially, often bilaterally, and thence to the iliac nodes.

Symptoms

The earliest symptom is usually pruritus; later a thickened area develops and this may ulcerate and bleed.

Treatment

Radical treatment is surgical—vulvectomy, with bilateral block dissection, unless the lesion is strictly unilateral or the patient is elderly. Vulval skin is relatively intolerant to irradiation, and radiotherapy at best is of only palliative value, except for radioactive needle implant to a very localised primary or recurrent lesion.

Results

Quoted results of treatment are up to 85% 5-year survival for early lesions, and 30–40% when lymph nodes are involved.

Choriocarcinoma

Trophoblastic tissue can undergo progressive cellular changes from simple hydropic degeneration, through hydatidiform mole and invasive mole, to choriocarcinoma. Hydatidiform mole shows some villous structures with little trophoblastic proliferation; invasive mole shows more trophoblastic activity with limited local invasion. Choriocarcinoma consists mainly of highly vascular anaplastic trophoblastic tissue.

Hydatidiform moles occur in about 1 in 2500 pregnancies, and choriocarcinoma in 1 in 30 000 in Europe; the incidence of the latter is much higher in Asia. About 50% of choriocarcinomas arise in moles; about 25% are preceded by spontaneous abortions and the other 25% occur after a normal or ectopic pregnancy.

It is suggested that abnormalities in the immunological defence mechanism of the mother are a factor in aetiology.

Local growth is rapid and metastases arise early, usually in the lungs. The tumour tissue produces human chorionic gonadotrophin (HCG), and estimation of the beta subgroup of this in the serum is of diagnostic and prognostic value.

Treatment

Emergency surgical treatment may be required to control bleeding; otherwise an attempt should be made to preserve uterine function. The uterus is evacuated by curettage initially; if there is residual disease, methotrexate therapy is given as most tumours are very sensitive to this. Thereafter, beta-HCG levels have usually fallen to within normal limits. Occasionally, hysterectomy is indicated for bulky residual disease. Follow-up is continued for 2 years, and if no recurrence is demonstrable a further pregnancy can be safely undertaken.

Methotrexate is a highly effective agent and other forms of chemotherapy seldom are needed; a possible second line regimen is actinomycin-D, vincristine and cyclophosphamide in combination. Local radiotherapy is seldom indicated. Rarely, spontaneous regression occurs.

Results

Treatment results in prolonged complete regression rates of about 90%; even in the presence of distant metastases with massive lung infiltration or CNS invasion, figures of 45–75% are quoted. Most of these patients are cured; relapses after 1 year are rare.

Male genital tract

Testis

The majority of testicular tumours are malignant, but they account for less than 1% of all cancers. Their incidence is 2 or 3 per 100 000 males per year.

They may be classified as in Table 10.3.

Seminomas account for about 75% of adult tumours, teratomas for about 20%, and the others for the remaining 5%. About 10% of teratomas show a seminomatous element. Teratoma may arise in childhood, most often in an undescended testis, and tending to be less malignant than in the adult.

Interstitial cell tumours are commonest about puberty; they may have marked virilising effects; about 90% are benign. Sertoli cell tumours are uncommon; they may secrete large amounts of oestrogen and produce gynaecomastia: they usually are benign. These tumours are treated surgically.

Lymphomas of the testis occur mainly in elderly men. Not infrequently they are bilateral. They are managed as are lymphomas elsewhere.

Table 10.3. Classification of testicular tumours.

Seminoma—arising from the germinal epithelium of the seminiferous tubules
Teratoma
(a) Differentiated
(b) Malignant, intermediate
(c) Malignant, anaplastic
(d) Malignant, trophoblastic—arising from embryonic cells in the testis or
    from multipotential germ cells
Combined teratoma-seminoma
Interstitial cell tumour
Sertoli cell tumour—arising from glandular tissue
Malignant lymphoma
Fibrosarcoma $\Big\}$ arising from paratesticular tissue
Rhabdomyosarcoma

Fibrosarcoma of the spermatic cord and rhabdomyosarcoma of the tunica vaginalis tend to arise before the age of 20 years; they represent about 10% of testicular tumours in childhood. Fibrosarcomas are often well differentiated, and wide excision is usually adequate. Rhabdomyosarcomas are treated by a combination of excision, radiotherapy and cytotoxic therapy.

Incidence

The highest incidence of seminomas is in the third, fourth and fifth decades of life; that of teratomas is in the third and fourth decades. Both are slightly commoner on the right than the left, in the ratio 5 : 4, except when they arise in an undescended testis when the incidence is equal. Occasionally they occur bilaterally (2 or 3% of tumours).

Predisposing factors and behaviour

Of possible predisposing factors the best established is non-descent or maldescent of the organ. The incidence of malignancy in an inguinal testis is about 1 in 80; for an intra-abdominal testis it is about 1 in 20. If an inguinal testis can be secured in the scrotum by operation (orchidopexy) before puberty, the risk of malignancy is reduced to that for a normal testis.

Injury is blamed (by the patient) in some cases, but there is no statistically significant evidence for this; injury may merely draw attention to a previously existing tumour. There may be a past history of mumps orchitis, but likewise this is not relevant.

Occasionally, a testicular tumour is associated with an hydrocele. There is an increased incidence of infertility or subfertility in association with testicular tumours.

Seminomas spread mainly via the lymphatics; teratomas have a greater tendency to haematogenous dissemination. The main lymphatic channels from the testis pass to the para-aortic nodes at the level of the renal arteries, but colateral spread can lead to iliac node involvement. Drainage to the inguinal nodes is only from the scrotum.

Some testicular tumours, especially teratomas, secrete marker substances. Chorionic gonadotrophin may be demonstrable in the urine, and also in the blood (as beta-HCG), and alpha-fetoprotein may be present in excess in the blood. The presence of these hormones or proteins may be of diagnostic value, and serial estimations can be of great value in follow-up monitoring.

Symptoms

The cardinal symptom is the presence of a mass—in about 80% of cases. Usually this is painless but a sense of heaviness is common. Occasionally, the presenting symptoms are referable to metastases. There may be local redness and tenderness suggesting an inflammatory lesion.

Investigations

Investigations include chest X-ray films (PA and lateral), CT scanning, bilateral lower limb lymphography combined with intravenous pyelography, urine hormone assays and blood beta-HCG and alpha-fetoprotein assays. Sperm count may be of value in assessing basic fertility.

Treatment

The initial treatment of all testicular tumours is orchidectomy. This removes the primary tumour, and provides the pathologist with the best possible material for an accurate histological diagnosis. Seminomas are very radiosensitive; the ipsilateral and central pelvic nodes, together with the para-aortic nodes, are irradiated. Teratomas are much more radioresistant, and a higher dose is needed; because of their tendency to metastasise early cytotoxic chemotherapy often becomes the primary treatment.

Metastases of seminoma in the chest can be treated by chest baths, with additional treatment to the mediastinum and supraclavicular areas. If the lungs are clear radiologically the latter areas only can be irradiated. Spread of teratoma to the supraclavicular fossae or mediastinum only may respond to full dose treatment, but if the lungs are involved chemotherapy is indicated. Usually, the remaining testis is not directly irradiated.

Because seminomas are so radiosensitive chemotherapy is seldom needed. However, responses to previously available agents were very poor. Much better responses are now achieved with newer agents such as cisplatin and etoposide.

For teratomas, a combination of vinblastine bolus injections with infusions of bleomycin was popular and of some value as palliation. Recently this has been superseded by combinations of vinblastine, bleomycin, cisplatin and etoposide, early results from which are encouraging. Trophoblastic teratomas are treated with vincristine and high-dose methotrexate with folinic acid rescue.

Results

The results of treatment of seminomas are good. In early cases, orchidectomy and radiotherapy to the pelvic and para-aortic nodes yields 5-year survival figures of about 85%, and few cases show evidence of recurrence or metastases after 3 years. For teratomas the corresponding figure is about 50%; good results are being achieved with chemotherapy.

Prostate

The commonest prostatic tumour is the adenocarcinoma. Its highest incidence is in the elderly. It may be found incidentally in glands removed for 'simple hypertrophy' causing urinary obstruction. After lung and bowel cancer in males it is the next most commonly fatal cancer, accounting for about 7% of cancer deaths.

It may present with gradually increasing difficulty in micturition, as local pain, or as pain from distant metastases (usually in bone). Local spread is to the bladder and rectum, and pelvic lymph nodes; later the para-aortic nodes may be involved. Blood spread is not uncommon. Bone metastases often are of sclerotic (osteoblastic) type.

The prostate secretes an enzyme, acid phosphatase, which can be measured in the blood, and which may be present in excess in prostatic carcinoma. It may be of value in diagnosis and in monitoring response to treatment.

The gland is normally under hormonal control, and adenocarcinomas may show a response to orchidectomy, or the administration of exogenous oestrogens (e.g. stilboestrol, ethinyloestradiol), or of fosfestrol, which is activated by the enzyme acid phosphatase to produce stilboestrol. The anti-androgen cyproterone is also under evaluation as palliative therapy. Radical treatment is prostatectomy, but many patients are too old and frail or the disease is too advanced for this. Radiotherapy to the primary tumour is of limited value, but can be effective in the treatment of painful bony deposits.

Overall 5-year survival is about 40%.

Penis

Malignant disease of the penis rarely, if ever, occurs in males circumcised in infancy, suggesting that hygienic factors are important in causation. Tumours, almost always squamous cell carcinomas, arise most commonly on the glans, but occasionally on the shaft of the organ. The incidence is high in Asiatic countries (up to 20% of all cancers), but is low in Europe (about 5%).

Many patients are elderly, with a limited life expectancy, and for infiltrating lesions of the middle and distal thirds surgical amputation is simple and safe, and effective. For younger patients, radical radiotherapy may be chosen by the patient; it can be curative and amputation still is available for residual or recurrent local disease.

Lymphatic spread is to the inguinal nodes, and operable deposits require radical block dissection; otherwise local radiotherapy may be of some value.

In the absence of groin node deposits the 5-year survival figures are about 90%; if local nodes are involved the figure falls to about 50%.

Urinary tract

Kidney

Malignant tumours of the kidney include hypernephroma (renal adenocarcinoma) and Wilm's tumour (nephroblastoma). Wilm's tumour is considered in Chapter 12.

Hypernephroma is thought to arise from the epithelium of the renal tubules. It is commonest in the sixth and seventh decades of life, and occurs in males twice as frequently as in females. The tumour often grows silently until locally advanced or until distant metastases are evident, for example a pathological fracture through a bony deposit. Some present early with haematuria, loin pain or episodes of pyrexia. Rarely, it is associated with polycythaemia.

Local extension into the renal vein is common, hence the high incidence of metastases in bones, lungs and brain. Local invasion of the perinephric fat and other adjacent structures occurs, and the para-aortic lymph nodes may become involved.

Investigations

Investigations include full blood count, plasma urea and electrolyte estimations, microscopical examination of the centrifuged deposit of the urine (for red blood corpuscles), chest X-ray films, CT scanning, radiological and radioisotopic skeletal surveys, intravenous pyelography, retrograde pyelography, renal arteriography, ultrasonography and radioisotope renography. The IVP may show a space-occupying lesion in the kidney, and this may be confirmed by retrograde pyelography. Renal arteriography can show an abnormal tumour circulation, which can be diagnostic.

Treatment

Hypernephroma is relatively radioresistant, and the only curative treatment is surgical excision of the kidney and its contained tumour. Postoperative radiotherapy to the renal bed has been claimed as of some value for locally advanced tumours, but is of little value as the sole means of treatment. Local palliative irradiation of isolated bony metastases may be helpful. Cytotoxic chemotherapy is ineffective.

Some tumours and their metastases, in males more often than in females, show limited responses to progestogen therapy, for example medroxyprogesterone, in high dosage. This may be related to the common embryological origin of the kidney and uterus from the nephrogenital ridge, the uterus being very sensitive to progestogens.

Results

Quoted survival figures are:
    Low-grade tumours—86% at 5 years; 60% at 10 years.
    High-grade tumours—29% at 5 years; 18% at 10 years.
Hypernephroma is a tumour which can manifest distant metastases many years after apparently successful treatment of the primary, hence the much lower 10-year figures as compared with those at 5 years.

Renal pelvis and ureter

These can be considered together. Tumours are rare, and have their highest incidence in the sixth and seventh decades of life. There are two histological types, transitional cell carcinoma and squamous cell carcinoma. The former is more common than the latter. The transitional cell carcinoma occurs more frequently in males than in females in the ratio 4 : 1; the squamous cell carcinoma shows an equal sex incidence.

These tumours are relatively radioresistant, and surgical excision is the treatment of choice. For locally invasive tumours, high-dose radiotherapy may be of some value as an adjunct to surgery, but is of little value as the sole mode of treatment.

Five-year survival figures for localised tumours exceed 50%; for tumours which have invaded local tissues the figure is much lower.

Adrenal gland

This is a convenient point at which to mention tumours of the adrenal gland, although they are not related functionally to the urogenital tract.

Neuroblastoma

Neuroblastoma is considered in Chapter 12, with other tumours of child-hood.

Adrenocortical tumours

About one-quarter of cases of hypercortisolism are caused by tumours, approximately half of which are carcinomas (particularly in childhood). The resulting Cushing's syndrome is generally florid and rapidly pro-gressive. Treatment of localised tumours is by surgery. Symptomatic relief in widespread or recurrent tumours may be achieved by drug therapy, for example with metyrapone or aminoglutethimide.

Adrenocortical tumours may also be responsible for virilising or feminis-ing syndromes, the latter much less commonly than the former, sometimes in combination with features of Cushing's syndrome. Treatment is again by surgery where possible. Hyperaldosteronism (Conn's syndrome) resulting from an aldosteronoma of the zona glomerulosa responds well to surgical excision of the tumour which usually is benign. Patients unsuit-able for operation are treated with spironolactone, an aldosterone antagon-ist, often very effectively.

Phaeochromocytoma is discussed in Chapter 16.

Bladder

Malignant tumours of the urinary bladder account for about 3% of cancers, but the incidence is rising, probably because of the excretion of environmental carcinogens in the urine.

Certainly some chemical agents are highly carcinogenic, for example beta-naphthylamine used in the dye industry, and certain other hydrocarbons used in the rubber and cable industries. There is an association between bladder cancer and bilharzia, a water-borne disease caused by a schistosome (*Schistosoma haematobium*) which is prevalent in Egypt. Malignant change in a benign papilloma is also a factor in aetiology. It is suggested that tars in tobacco smoke may be excreted in the urine and may be carcinogenic to the bladder mucosa.

Incidence and symptoms

The peak incidence is in the seventh decade of life, and males are affected three times as commonly as females. Epithelial tumours range from benign papillomas to invasive transitional cell carcinomas. The former may be single or multiple. The latter show all grades from well-differentiated to poorly differentiated (anaplastic) tumours. Occasionally, squamous cell carcinomas and adenocarcinomas are reported. Rarely, benign or malignant connective tissue tumours occur, and rhabdomyosarcoma of the bladder can arise in childhood. However, about 99% of tumours are of epithelial origin. The cardinal symptom is haematuria.

Investigations

Cystoscopy and biopsy, and pelvic examination under anaesthesia are essential in the diagnosis and assessment of the primary tumour. Other investigations include assessment of renal function, cytological examination of the centrifuged deposit of the urine, lymphography, and intravenous pyelography. The latter is especially important as a bladder tumour may be secondary to a tumour higher in the urinary tract.

Treatment

Small superficial well-differentiated tumours, single or multiple, benign or malignant, can be treated by perurethral diathermy, followed by careful and frequent cystoscopic examination, so that any recurrence or new tumours can be detected early and treated. Multiple tumours may require several sessions of treatment. Infiltrating and poorly differentiated tumours are best treated by radiotherapy followed by total cystectomy. Radiotherapy is by beam directed high-energy techniques. It is a strenuous treatment, often causing temporary increased frequency and dysuria, and diarrhoea and tenesmus. A high fluid intake should be maintained, urinary antiseptics or antibiotics should be prescribed as appropriate, and antidiarrhoeal drugs may be needed. For poorly differentiated multiple tumours total cystectomy is indicated as the definitive treatment.

Some authorities advocate partial cystectomy for infiltrating, but localised, tumours away from the trigone area, and for tumours of the vault or in association with a diverticulum. In the past, radioactive gold grain implants have been used for well-differentiated, solitary, superficial tumours not amenable to perurethral diathermy, but this technique is falling out of favour. Intravesical installation of chemotherapeutic agents (particularly Epodyl, an epoxide with alkylating properties) for numerous superficial tumours has its advocates, and colloidal radioactive gold-198 has been similarly used.

Palliative radiotherapy is of limited value. Bladder carcinomas are not very radiosensitive and the upset from treatment of sufficient dose to achieve any response may be more distressing than the benefits obtained.

Long-term follow-up, clinically and cystoscopically, is essential. Late effects of radiotherapy include contraction of the bladder, and telangiectases of the mucosa which may produce haematuria.

Results

Early superficial tumours show a 5-year survival rate of about 75%; for tumours which have invaded the muscle of the bladder wall the figure is about 50%; tumours through the full thickness of the wall show about 20% 5-year survival; extravesical extension reduces the figure to about 10%.

Urethra

Malignant tumours of the urethra are rare. Most are squamous carcinomas; a few are of transitional cell type.

Their site, apart from tumours of the penile urethra, makes surgical treatment difficult without total cystectomy and implantation of the ureters into an ileal loop conduit; radiotherapy is usually therefore needed. Radioactive needle implant for localised tumours of the female urethra may be effective both therapeutically and functionally. Otherwise, small field beam directed treatment is indicated.

For early lesions 5-year survival of about 50% has been reported.

Chapter 11
Haemopoietic and Lymphoreticular Malignancies

The malignancies derived from cells of the bone marrow and lymphoreticular system comprise mainly the leukaemias, the lymphomas and myeloma. A more complete list is given in Table 11.1. These neoplasms account for less than 10% of all malignant disease, but are important because many are now known to be curable by newer techniques of radiotherapy and particularly cytotoxic chemotherapy.

Table 11.1. Myelo-, lympho- and immunoproliferative diseases.

LEUKAEMIAS
Acute
  Lymphoblastic
  Non-lymphoblastic ·
  (a) Myeloblastic
  (b) Promyeloblastic
  (c) Myelomonocytic, monocytic
  (d) Erythroleukaemia
Chronic
  Lymphocytic
  Myeloid (granulocytic)

POLYCYTHAEMIA VERA

LYMPHOMAS
Hodgkin's disease
Non-Hodgkin's lymphoma

MYELOMA

WALDENSTRÖM'S MACROGLOBULINAEMIA

HEAVY CHAIN DISEASE

OTHERS
Leukaemic reticuloendotheliosis
Malignant histiocytosis
Mastocytosis

Polycythaemia vera is a proliferative, not strictly speaking a neoplastic, disorder; it is included here for completeness.

Leukaemia

The leukaemias are malignant neoplasms of leucopoeitic cells and are classified according to the cell type which predominates. The acute leukaemias are now recognised to be heterogenous diseases; acute lymphoblastic leukaemia is most common in childhood but after early adulthood acute non-lymphoblastic leukaemia is commoner. The investigation and management of acute lymphoblastic leukaemia in the adult is similar to that in the child (see Chapter 12) though the prognosis is worse. Acute non-lymphoblastic leukaemia includes myeloblastic leukaemia, by far the commonest, and the promyelocytic, myelomonocytic and monocytic types and erythroleukaemia.

Acute myeloblastic leukaemia

Acute myeloblastic leukaemia, maximum incidence at 40–60 years, is characterised by replacement of normal bone marrow cells by primitive cells giving anaemia, thrombocytopenia and depletion of normal leucocytes; other tissues, for example spleen, liver and lymph nodes, are involved less frequently than in acute lymphoblastic leukaemia.

Clinical presentation

The clinical presentation is therefore of a short history of generalised malaise, anaemia, bleeding diathesis (particularly purpura and bleeding gums) and infection. Occasionally splenomegaly and lymphadenopathy are present.

Diagnosis

The diagnosis is confirmed by examination of peripheral blood films and bone marrow aspirate. The use of differential staining techniques (PAS, Sudan black, peroxidase), cytogenetic studies (bone marrow chromosomal abnormalities are seen in about one-half of cases and may differ according to the type of leukaemia), and electronmicroscopy aids the accurate classification of the leukaemia in most cases.

Certain patients, particularly adult males, present with 'preleukaemia'— a smouldering condition in which there is refractory pancytopenia, with some evidence of abnormal primitive cells in the blood and/or bone marrow.

Eventually the condition develops into florid leukaemia and conventional treatment is necessary.

Treatment

The treatment of acute myeloblastic leukaemia has not shown the significant improvement in outlook seen in acute lymphoblastic leukaemia. Remission induction is attempted using a drug combination such as cytosine arabinoside, thioguanine and daunorubicin. Prolonged myelosuppression may result after this therapy and severe infection is a major limiting factor in trying to achieve complete haematological remission. Supportive measures include prophylactic antibiotics, the use of an isolated protected environment, aggressive treatment of infections, and the appropriate administration of granulocyte transfusions.

Maintenance therapy usually involves the further periodic administration of intensive chemotherapy, often of the type used in the induction regimen. Meningeal involvement in myeloblastic leukaemia is uncommon; on current evidence prophylactic CNS therapy is not warranted. When relapse occurs very few patients attain second remission even with alternative intensive therapy. Immunotherapy, using either non-specific stimulation (e.g. with BCG) or with irradiated allogeneic myeloblasts, has proved generally disappointing.

The treatment of acute leukaemia has recently been revolutionised by the introduction of bone marrow transplantation. This involves the transfer of a viable population of myelopoietic and lymphopoietic stem cells. The vast majority of bone marrow transplants are performed between major histocompatibility complex identical sibling pairs (allogeneic transplantation). Bone marrow transplantation has been used mainly in patients with acute myeloid leukaemia either in their first remission after chemotherapy or at relapse, and in acute lymphoblastic leukaemia where there is a high risk of relapse after remission or where the disease is refractory to chemotherapy regimens. The actual procedure involves the administration of high-dose chemotherapy followed a couple of days later by total body irradiation. The bone marrow is harvested from the donor from multiple bone marrow punctures under general anaesthetic and then transfused into the patient after his myelo-ablative therapy. The procedure may be complicated by graft v. host disease, which may be either acute or chronic, and immunosuppressive therapy is therefore given. Corticosteroids and methotrexate have traditionally been used, but more recently cyclosporin A, which has a selective inhibitory effect on T cells, has been successfully introduced. Such patients are of course very prone to infection and need to be nursed in as sterile an environment as can be managed.

Prophylactic anti-fungal agents are often given, together with non-absorbable antibiotics, to sterilize the gastrointestinal tract. It has recently been suggested that co-trimoxazole and acyclovir should be given as prophylaxis against pneumocystis and herpes infections respectively. Cytomegalovirus remains a serious problem, and as yet there is no treatment for this.

Prognosis

The prognosis is improving, though it is still rather poor especially in older patients. Remission can be induced in most patients but relapse is common and median survival is between 9 and 18 months, though long-term survival, of the order 10–20%, is possible.

Other acute non-lymphoblastic leukaemias

Other acute non-lymphoblastic leukaemias are investigated and treated in much the same way as acute myeloblastic leukaemia. The monocytic varieties may present insidiously over many months before accurate diagnosis. They tend to occur in middle life; oral ulceration and swelling of the gums are special features. Acute promyelocytic leukaemia is not uncommonly complicated by disseminated intravascular coagulation as the leukaemic cell granules release fibrinolytic substances.

Acute erythroleukaemia

Acute erythroleukaemia (Di Guglielmo's syndrome, erythraemic myelosis) is usually an acute rapidly progressive disease involving neoplastic proliferation of erythroid and myeloid cells and presenting with anaemia, fever and splenomegaly. It commonly terminates in acute myeloblastic leukaemia.

Chronic myeloid (granulocytic) leukaemia

This type of leukaemia, accounting for up to a quarter of human leukaemias, occurs chiefly between the ages of 15 and 40. Most patients have a distinct chromosomal abnormality in their haemopoietic cells; this is called the Philadelphia (Ph[1]) chromosome, in which there is a deletion of the long arm of the chromosome 22 pair.

Clinical presentation

The clinical presentation is classically of splenomegaly with its associated symptoms, or of chronic ill health with anaemia and bleeding abnormalities; the disorder may also be a chance finding.

Diagnosis

The diagnosis is suggested by finding a raised peripheral white blood cell count (often above $100 \times 10^9/1$) with identification of immature cells of the granulocyte series, mainly promyelocytes and myelocytes; bone marrow examination confirms the diagnosis. The platelet count may be elevated and the haemoglobin normal or low normal. The differential diagnosis includes polycythaemia vera, myelofibrosis and the 'leukaemoid' reaction to infection or metastatic malignancy. The Ph^1 chromosome is not present in these conditions, however, and the leucocyte alkaline phosphatase is generally increased, whereas in chronic myeloid leukaemia it is nearly always decreased.

Over the first three or so years of the disease more mature myeloid cells predominate in the blood. After this time, however, a transformation usually takes place (blast cell crisis) and more primitive cells become evident.

Treatment

The treatment of chronic myeloid leukaemia in its early phases has traditionally been by administration of continuous busulphan therapy. More recently combination chemotherapy (e.g. with thioguanine plus busulphan or more intensive regimens and splenectomy) has been tried and results of controlled trials are awaited.

Despite treatment progression of the disease is invariable; the spleen may become massive, and refractory anaemia and increased susceptibility to infection are problems. Splenic irradiation may palliate the massive splenomegaly; infections must be identified and treated vigorously.

Even with current chemotherapeutic regimens the prognosis is poor and the inevitable transformation (blastic crisis) is still usually a terminal event; survival at this stage can be measured in weeks or months. The median survival time of chronic myeloid leukaemia from presentation is 3–4 years.

Chronic lymphocytic leukaemia

This is the commonest type of leukaemia and is typically a disorder of older age, most patients being over the age of 50 years. There is a male preponderance and the clinical manifestations are those produced by greatly increased numbers of apparently mature long-lived lymphocytes, usually of B cell type, in the blood, bone marrow and lymphoreticular tissues.

Clinical presentation

The classical presentation is of generalised lymphadenopathy with spleno-megaly. Less often the disease is a chance finding on routine investigation or presents as a result of infection (due to impaired humoral immunity with hypogammaglobulinaemia), or as anaemia, thrombocytopenia or generalised malaise.

Diagnosis

The diagnosis is confirmed by finding that the peripheral white blood cell count is elevated with an increase of small mature lymphocytes. Anaemia may occur as a result of marrow infiltration, or autoimmune Coombs' test positive haemolytic anaemia—a not uncommon finding in this disorder—or of hypersplenism secondary to splenomegaly. Bone marrow examination shows replacement by lymphocytes similar to those seen in the blood.

Treatment

Treatment of this disorder depends on the clinical assessment of the patient and of the nature of the disease. It is recognised that many patients remain asymptomatic for many years without treatment; in others downhill progress may be rapid. Most authorities treat if the patient has symptoms or if there is anaemia or profound thrombocytopenia. Radio-therapy may reduce the size of large gland masses or of a massive spleen, but the usual treatment is of continuous oral chlorambucil with or without prednisolone. Sometimes the disease behaves more aggressively and in such cases combination chemotherapy may be appropriate.

Prognosis

The prognosis in chronic lymphocytic leukaemia is generally good, despite the broad spectrum of the disorder, with a median survival time of over 5 years; death is usually by infection occuring as a result of the defective humoral immune response.

Polycythaemia vera

This is a myeloproliferative disorder characterised by the benign prolifer-ation of haemopoietic cells; myeloid metaplasia and idiopathic thrombo-cythaemia are related variants. In polycythaemia vera erythroid precursors are primarily involved, though there is increased activity of white cell and platelet precursors. There is an increase in the number of circulating erythrocytes and an increase in red cell volume; usually there is also leucocytosis and thrombocytosis (often with platelet dysfunction). It is commoner in males than females and has its highest incidence in the sixth and seventh decades of life.

Clinical presentation

The clinical presentation relates to the effects of hyperviscosity, hyper-volaemia and coagulation abnormalities. The commonest symptoms arise from the central nervous system (headaches, dizziness, vertigo) and cardio-vascular system (heart failure, thrombotic episodes, abnormal bleeding). Pruritus and gout (from secondary hyperuricaemia) may be found. The patient is often plethoric and cyanosed; splenomegaly and slight hepatomegaly are common.

Diagnosis

Diagnostic findings include an increased haematocrit and red cell volume, normal arterial blood gases (to differentiate it from hypoxic polycythaemia), hyperactive bone marrow and increased marrow iron turnover.

Treatment

Treatment is aimed at reducing the red cell volume. This can be achieved by repeated venesection, which gives only short-lived benefit and may be technically difficult because of the tendency of blood to clot during the procedure, by chemotherapy, usually intermittent busulphan, chloram-bucil, hydroxyurea or melphalan, or by administration of radioactive phos-phorus (^{32}P) which emits beta-rays and destroys myelo-proliferating cells.

Prognosis

The prognosis is undoubtedly improved by therapy; without treatment the median survival is about 5 years, with treatment it is 10 years.

About 10% of patients develop terminal acute leukaemia. In most of the others the disease follows a clinical course resembling myelofibrosis; the spleen enlarges markedly, the marrow becomes hypocellular and refractory pancytopenia results.

Malignant lymphoma

Malignant lymphoma is divided into two groups of diseases—Hodgkin's disease and non-Hodgkin's lymphoma. The former has fairly well-standardised histology typing, staging criteria and treatment protocols; the latter is still the subject of much international debate and standardised investigation and management indices have not yet been universally established.

Hodgkin's disease

Hodgkin's disease, first described by Sir Thomas Hodgkin in 1832, is in most countries the commonest malignant lymphoma; in the United Kingdom it has an incidence of 3–4 cases per 100 000 population per year. The disease has a bimodal age incidence, one peak occurring at 15–34 years and the other after 50 years; it is generally commoner in males than females.

Aetiology

The aetiology of Hodgkin's disease is unknown. There is some evidence for the infective 'spread' of Hodgkin's disease in the community and there is a twofold increased risk in the relatives of patients. Time–space clustering of cases is well established, but evidence such as this for a viral aetiology in young patients is still circumstantial. The origin of the tumour from immune cells has led to the theory that Hodgkin's disease is immunologically mediated either by a continuous antigen challenge mechanism or by failure of the innate immunological 'surveillance' system; again there is no convincing evidence to support this. Environmental factors have also been incriminated, but it seems likely on present knowledge that the cause is multifactorial.

Histology

The Rye classification is generally used to differentiate the histological types of Hodgkin's disease:
1 Lymphocyte predominant.
2 Nodular sclerosis.
3 Mixed cellularity.
4 Lymphocyte depletion.
 The key cell in the diagnosis is the Reed–Sternberg cell; classically this is a 'mirror image' binucleate large cell but its identification is not always

straightforward. Other cells including lymphocytes, histiocytes, plasma cells, eosinophils and fibroblasts are also seen in diseased tissue.

The most frequent histological type seen is the nodular sclerosis variety. The next most frequent is the mixed cellularity type—it occurs in all age groups and in all forms of presentation. Lymphocyte-predominant histology, with its plentiful normal lymphocytes, perhaps implying a good immune response to the tumour, is usually seen in young adults and neck presentations. Lymphocyte-depletion histology, the other end of the spectrum, is seen in older age groups. The nodular sclerosis variety can be subtyped into good and bad grades depending on the background cellular make-up. It is usually seen in young patients and is often associated with mediastinal gland involvement.

Clinical presentation and investigation

The classical clinical presentation (two-thirds of cases) is of neck lymphadenopathy. Less frequently (15–20%) groin or axillary nodes are first involved. Sometimes the lymphadenopathy is generalised or the patient may present with systemic symptoms. Rarely, structures outside the lymphatic system (extranodal sites) are primarily involved. As the disease advances multiple lymphatic and extralymphatic (e.g. liver, bone, bone marrow, lung, kidneys etc.) sites may be involved.

The disease is investigated and staged at presentation by the Ann Arbor criteria (Table 11.2 and Fig. 11.1); from stage 1–4 and A or B.

The main differential diagnosis of chronic lymphadenopathy in the younger patient is infection (e.g. ongoing regional sepsis, viral infections,

Table 11.2. The Ann Arbor staging criteria.

Stage 1 Single lymph node region involved
Stage 2 Two or more lymph node regions involved but on the same side of the diaphragm
Stage 3 Involvement of lymph node regions on both sides of the diaphragm
Stage 4 Generalised involvement of one or more extralymphatic organs with or without lymph node disease

Localised extralymphatic lesions with or without associated lymph node involvement are termed 'E' (extranodal) lesions

Category A Asymptomatic
Category B Symptomatic

i.e. weight loss (> 10% of body weight in prior 6 months), unexplained persistent fever; night sweats

---

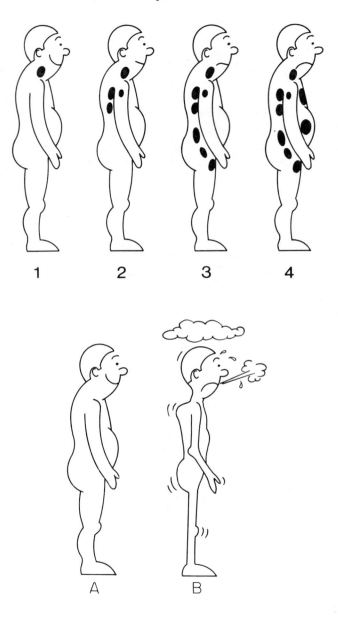

Fig. 11.1. The Ann Arbor staging for malignant lymphoma.

toxoplasmosis, brucellosis), but sarcoidosis and 'immunological' lymph-adenopathy (e.g. with collagen vascular diseases) are sometimes a problem. In the older patient it is important to remember that the commonest cause of localised lymphadenopathy is secondary carcinoma, and of generalised lymphadenopathy is chronic lymphocytic leukaemia.

The three constitutional symptoms of relevance to the 'B' category are weight loss, abnormal (usually nocturnal) sweating and persistent pyrexia, occasionally of the undulant Pel–Ebstein variety. Pruritus and alcohol-induced pain in diseased tissue are non-specific, though important symptoms. Full clinical examination is followed by histological examination of an adequate tissue biopsy and then by investigation. A full peripheral blood count and film is mandatory. Lymphopenia, neutrophilia and eosinophilia are all features of more widespread disease; the ESR may also provide a guide as to the severity of the disease. Biochemical investigations include hepatic and renal function tests though it must be realised that extensive involvement of liver and kidneys can occur before such tests become abnormal. Immunological investigations to assess T and B cell function are also helpful—depressed immunity tends to be a feature of widespread disease. Isotope scanning of the liver (to assess particularly infiltration) and the spleen (to assess particularly the size) are important, and chest radiography with appropriate tomography is vital to detect the mediastinal and hilar lymphadenopathy found in up to a quarter of patients. Though CT scanning is playing an increasingly important role, lymphography is established in the staging procedure of Hodgkin's disease; characteristically the diseased nodes look large and foamy but these appearances are non-specific and must be taken in conjunction with the clinical and pathological findings. The oily contrast often remains in the nodes for many months; serial follow-up films are therefore very important. Lymphography is often followed by intravenous pyelography; displacement of the ureters and renal abnormalities are occasionally found. Since lymphography does not demonstrate abnormalities in the upper para-aortic and mesenteric nodes, ultrasound and CT scanning of this region can be extremely useful. Other investigations are selected on clinical judgment, for example skeletal X-rays and isotope scans, gastrointestinal (barium) radiography.

Over the past few years it has been realised that intra-abdominal involvement with lymphoma may accompany apparently isolated superficial lymphadenopathy remote from the abdomen. The clinical assessment of liver and spleen involvement by lymphoma is notoriously difficult; the clinically large spleen found in up to one-third of cases may, for example, show only reactive or granulomatous changes and the normal sized spleen may show pathological evidence of disease. For these reasons diagnostic laparotomy with splenectomy and liver, lymph node and bone marrow biopsy is now acknowledged to play a part in the staging of selected patients with Hodgkin's disease. Removal of the spleen also has the advantage of obviating the need to irradiate that area, with subsequent radiation damage to the left kidney and left lung base. It has the disadvantage, apart from the operative morbidity, of possibly making the patient more prone to infections, particularly septicaemia.

If laparatomy is performed the patient is restaged according to the pathological findings.

Treatment

The treatment of localised Hodgkin's disease is primarily by fractionated radical mega-voltage wide field radiotherapy. Areas adjacent to involved sites are often irradiated prophylactically. The standard fields are called Mantle (covering the neck, thoracic and axillary node areas) and Inverted Y (covering the femoral, inguinal, iliac and para-aortic node areas). Total nodal irradiation, i.e. Mantle followed by Inverted Y (or vice versa), may be given for intermediate stages of the disease; but the treatment for widespread lymphoma is cyclical combination chemotherapy. The classical regimen is MOPP—Mustine, Oncovin (vincristine), prednisolone, procarbazine; other regimens include ABVD—Adriamycin (doxorubicin), bleomycin, Velbe (vinblastine), DTIC (dacarbazine); ABCP—Adriamycin, bleomycin, CCNU, prednisolone; and LOPP—Leukeran (chlorambucil), Oncovin, prednisolone, procarbazine. A promising development has been the successful use of alternating cycles of non-cross resistant drugs (e.g. MOPP/ABVD).

One of the commonest problems in the treatment of Hodgkin's disease, particularly when chemotherapy is used, is infection, usually with Herpes zoster or *Candida albicans,* but occasionally with bacteria (e.g. septicaemia) or opportunists (e.g. *Pneumocystis, Aspergillus, Cryptococcus*).

Prognosis

The prognosis in Hodgkin's disease has improved considerably over the past two decades. Suffice to say that with localised disease treated by radical irradiation in specialised centres at least 80% 5-year disease-free survival is now the rule; with widespread disease treated by cytotoxic chemotherapy 5-year disease-free survivals of at least 40–50% are possible.

The prognostic importance of age (young patients do better than old), sex (females fare better than males), histological type (certain features, e.g. lymphocyte predominance, are associated with good prognosis; others, e.g. mixed cellularity/lymphocyte depletion, are less favourable), clinical stage and symptom status (localised asymptomatic disease tends to do well, generalised symptomatic disease does not) must always be kept in mind when assessing the likely response to therapy.

There is no evidence that either pregnancy or the treatment with hormonal preparations (e.g. the contraceptive pill) adversely affects Hodgkin's disease or other lymphomas.

Non-Hodgkin's lymphoma

Non-Hodgkin's lymphoma refers to a heterogenous group of disorders with varying clinical presentations and histological findings. Generally the prognosis in this group is worse than in Hodgkin's disease; this seems to be particularly so for children. The maximum incidence is between 50–70 years of age with only a slight male preponderance; the overall incidence is about 2–3 cases per 100 000 per year.

Immunological factors may be important aetiologically—an increased incidence of these tumours has been reported in immunosuppressed organ transplant patients, in congenital immunodeficiency syndromes and with autoimmune disease.

Clinical presentation

The clinical presentation is similar to that of Hodgkin's disease but the lymphadenopathy is more often generalised and tends to be centrifugal, so that epitrochlear, mesenteric, nasopharyngeal (Waldeyer's ring) and intestinal (Peyer's patches) lymphatic tissue may be involved. Extranodal disease occurs more frequently than in Hodgkin's disease. Primary lymphoma of extranodal tissues, particularly gut, nasopharynx, bone (found in younger age groups) and skin is well recognised. These features emphasise the multifocal nature of non-Hodgkin's lymphoma as opposed to the often contiguous nature of Hodgkin's disease. Systemic symptoms, identical to those in Hodgkin's disease, occur in up to a quarter of patients at presentation.

Histology

The histological sub-classification of non-Hodgkin's lymphoma is controversial. The terms lymphosarcoma, reticulum cell sarcoma and giant follicular lymphoma are now largely redundant. Most newer classifications recognise the importance of dividing these lymphomas into nodular (or follicular) and diffuse types and thereafter to define the cell type involved. The early Rappaport classification divided the cell types basically into lymphocytic (small and large), histiocytic (reticulum cell) and mixed. More recent classifications have defined non-Hodgkin's lymphoma according to functional origin (e.g. T cell, B, cell etc.) or according to purely morphological criteria. Most non-Hodgkin's lymphomas are of B cell type and arise from lymphocytes within the germinal follicles. Tumours from early follicle cells tend to form clusters (the so-called follicular pattern); these have a relatively good prognosis. Tumours from lymphocytes later in their follicular development or from immunoblasts show a more diffuse histological pattern and are more malignant in their behaviour. T cell lymphomas are relatively uncommon—these include mycosis fungoides, Sézary syndrome and a relatively malignant lymphoblastic lymphoma, often accompanied by leukaemia.

Of the many classifications of non-Hodgkin's lymphoma, the six best known have recently been compared by an international group, and a working formulation for clinical usage has been devised by which the various classifications may be harmonized. In this formulation lymphomas are grouped into low, intermediate and high-grade malignancy.

Investigations

The investigation of non-Hodgkin's lymphoma is aimed at staging the patient accurately, usually according to the Ann Arbor criteria (Fig. 11.1). The multifocal nature of the disease must be kept in mind. Particular investigative features of non-Hodgkin's lymphoma are the significant incidence of autoimmune haemolytic anaemia, the frequency (up to 15% at presentation) of bone marrow involvement and the occasional finding of monoclonal gammopathy on immunoglobulin assay. The place for exploratory laparotomy in non-Hodgkin's lymphoma is not yet established.

Treatment

In treatment it is important to take into account the patient's age and the histological type of the tumour, and to distinguish between extranodal, local nodal, regional nodal and generalised symptomatic disease. For the patient, particularly in the older age group, with lymphoma of favourable prognosis histology-type treatment may be palliative—this may involve local low-dose irradiation, single agent chemotherapy (chlorambucil + prednisolone) or nothing. Patients with more aggressive histological types with localised nodal or extranodal disease, respond well to local radical irradiation; this may also be appropriate for patients with regional disease though some authorities here advocate systemic therapy. For stage 3 and 4 disease, or for earlier stages with systemic symptoms, cyclical combination chemotherapy (e.g. with cyclophosphamide, vincristine, doxorubicin and prednisolone) is indicated.

There are many clinical studies now underway using intensive alternating (multiagent) regimens which obviously give better complete remission responses than the standard treatments, but at the expense of increased toxicity.

Prognosis

The prognosis varies enormously with histology and stage. For truly localised disease, survival rates of 60–80% disease-free at 5 years are possible; for widespread disease treated with chemotherapy the figures are 30–40%. Some non-Hodgkin's lymphomas can still, however, be inexorably fatal within a few weeks of presentation, irrespective of treatment.

Mycosis fungoides and Sézary syndrome

The majority of non-Hodgkin's lymphomas are believed to arise from B cells; of the T cell types mycosis fungoides and the Sézary syndrome, though both rare, are the most noteworthy. Mycosis fungoides describes a cutaneous lymphoma characteristically occurring in later life and progressing from non-specific 'premycotic' skin lesions to indurated skin plaques and then large nodules. The clinical course is classically one of slow disease progression, but over a period of time, sometimes years, lymphatic and visceral infiltration becomes a feature in most patients. Early skin lesions respond well to symptomatic treatment; in intermediate stages the lesions may respond to superficial irradiation, for example with electron beam therapy, or to psoralen and ultraviolet light therapy (PUVA). Advanced skin and systemic disease is difficult to treat though some short-term responses have been seen with combinations of cytotoxic agents; the median survival time in mycosis fungoides is about 5 years.

The Sézary syndrome describes a clinical and pathological entity, probably a variant of mycosis fungoides, in which erythroderma is combined with the presence of circulating abnormal T lymphocytes (Sézary cells). Disseminated lymphomatous lesions are found particularly in the terminal stages of the disease. Treatment is largely symptomatic.

Burkitt's lymphoma

Burkitt's lymphoma is a particular type of lymphoma found most commonly in tropical East Africa and believed to be aetiologically associated with a virus (the Epstein–Barr virus) acting in patients immunosuppressed by chronic malarial infection (see Chapter 1). It occurs classically in the age range 5–8 years and presents as single or multiple lymphatic tumours involving the jaw, gut, ovaries and testes. Central nervous system involvement, with spinal cord compression or basal meningeal infiltration is common. The classical histology is of an expanding mass of undifferentiated lymphoreticular cells containing numerous large macrophages producing the so-called 'starry sky' appearance. After staging of the disease the treatment is usually by chemotherapy (particularly with cyclophosphamide, vincristine and methotrexate) but relapse, even after long-term remission, is frequent. The overall survival is only about 30–40%.

Myeloma

Myelomatosis (multiple myeloma) is the commonest form of plasma cell neoplasm. The characteristic features of this chronic progressive disorder are due to infiltration of tissues, particularly bone marrow, by myeloma cells and to abnormal immunoglobulin production. The maximal incidence of the disease is in the age group 60–80 years. Solitary myeloma deposits (plasmacytomas) occasionally occur in the absence of evidence of overt disseminated disease.

The majority of solitary plasmacytomas of bone disseminate after a period as long as 20 years, giving rise to overt myelomatosis. A distinct, much rarer, entity is the extramedullary plasmacytoma most commonly found in upper respiratory tract tissues and behaving clinically like non-Hodgkin's lymphoma, of which it may be a variant. Myelomatosis rarely develops from the disorder, and treatment by surgery and radiotherapy is generally effective.

Clinical presentation

The clinical presentation of myelomatosis is protean. Symptoms result from bony lesions (pain, deformity, pathological fractures), from bone marrow infiltration (anaemia, haemorrhage) and from immunoglobulin abnormalities (infection). Nervous system pressure effects from myeloma deposits are not uncommon; spinal cord compression may result from a collapsed vertebrae. Chronic renal insufficiency is a common finding at some stage in the disease.

Diagnosis

The diagnosis is confirmed by satisfying two of the following three main criteria:

1 Bone marrow examination demonstrating abnormal infiltration by plasma cells.

2 Immunochemistry showing a protein abnormality.

3 Skeletal radiology showing bone lesions.

Haematological investigations invariably show some degree of anaemia and an elevated ESR. Protein electrophoresis demonstrates abnormal gammaglobulins; immunochemistry defines the nature of the gammopathy. The neoplastic proliferation of a single clone of cells gives rise to the production of a discrete monoclonal component or paraprotein. Excess light chains may be synthesised and appear in the urine as Bence-Jones protein. The paraprotein is produced at the expense of the other normal immunoglobulins which are therefore often reduced in level.

IgG myelomatosis accounts for over one-half and IgA myelomatosis for about a quarter of all cases. IgM, IgD and IgE myelomas are rare. Light chain (Bence-Jones protein) production alone is seen in the remaining cases. The abnormality must be differentiated from the benign monoclonal gammopathy of the elderly where the amount of paraprotein is small, does not increase with time and there is no evidence of systemic disease or of immunoparesis.

Skeletal radiology will reveal an abnormality in the majority of cases; osteolytic 'punched out' lesions are classical and they are often multiple, for example in the skull; in addition there may be pathological fractures or severe osteoporosis.

Biochemical assessment may demonstrate abnormal renal function, elevated serum calcium and, surprisingly, usually a normal alkaline phosphatase.

Renal insufficiency in myeloma is a bad prognostic sign and is one of the commonest causes of death from the disease. Contributing causes include hypercalcaemia, pyelonephritis, clotting abnormalities, proteinaceous tubular casts and amyloidosis.

Treatment

The treatment of myelomatosis is by cytotoxic chemotherapy and careful supportive measures. By using certain alkylating agents it is possible to improve the clinical status and increase survival times. Melphalan and cyclophosphamide have been commonly employed and intermittent high-dose regimens (e.g. melphalan and prednisolone) seem to be effective; multi-drug combination regimens have also shown good results. The importance of supportive therapy cannot be overemphasised; blood transfusion for anaemia, antibiotics for bacterial infections, plasmapheresis for hyperviscosity, and rehydration etc. for hypercalcaemia (see Chapter 16) all have a vital role to play. Radiotherapy to localised painful lesions is usually highly successful. Monitoring of response involves serial measurements of immunoglobulin and haemoglobin levels and of reassessing bone marrow infiltration.

Prognosis

The prognosis, though improved with chemotherapy, is still poor; the median survival of all patients is about 2 years, though in patients presenting early in the disease survival can be extended for several years by treatment. Bad prognostic features are uraemia, proteinuria, hypoalbuminaemia and severe anaemia.

Waldenström's macroglobulinaemia

This disease is a progressive systemic disorder in which lymphoid or plasmacytoid proliferation results in the production of a monoclonal IgM. It affects older people and shares the characteristics of both lymphoma and myeloma, with lymphoreticular and bone marrow involvement by abnormal cells; hyperviscosity with cerebral, cardiac or peripheral vascular insufficiency is a common finding, but bone involvement is rare. Treatment by chemotherapy (alkylating agent plus prednisolone) may give gratifying responses but the prognosis for survival is extremely variable—from a few months to several years. Plasmapheresis is important where there are symptoms indicative of hyperviscosity.

Heavy chain diseases

In these lymphoma-like immunoproliferative diseases there is a monoclonal production of anomalous heavy chains without light chains present. *Gamma* heavy chain disease occurs in older patients and resembles non-Hodgkin's lymphoma in clinical features; the Waldeyer's ring is frequently involved. *Alpha* heavy chain disease, so-called 'Mediterranean lymphoma', affects mainly the bowel in young adults and presents with diarrhoea, malabsorption and abdominal masses. *Mu* chain disease has been described in long-standing chronic lymphocytic leukaemia. In all types of disease the diagnosis is made by the immunochemical analysis of the abnormal protein. Treatment of these disorders is difficult though cytotoxic chemotherapy and radiotherapy may both have a part to play.

Other related disorders

Leukaemic reticuloendotheliosis (hairy cell leukaemia) is a rare condition usually affecting adult males and presenting with pancytopenia and splenomegaly. The hairy cells seen in the blood and involved tissues are probably neoplastic lymphocytes; they classically contain tartrate-resistant acid phosphatase. The prognosis is relatively good; chemotherapy rarely helps but splenectomy may lead to remission.

Malignant histiocytosis (histiocytic medullary reticulosis of Robb-Smith) is probably a rare variant of non-Hodgkin's lymphoma, characterised by a diffuse proliferation of abnormal histiocytes in lymphoreticular tissues. It is usually acute and rapidly progressive, and is usually fatal, rarely responding to chemotherapy.

Systemic mastocytosis is a rare progressive condition in which an abnormal proliferation of mast cells affects skin (as urticaria pigmentosa), viscera, bone and the entire reticuloendothelial system. Steroids may give temporary remission; other treatments have not proved beneficial.

Chapter 12
Childhood Tumours

After accidents tumours are the commonest cause of death in childhood. In a population of a million children (0–14 years of age) there will be about 100 new cases of malignancy each year.

In general paediatric tumours tend to be poorly differentiated, fast growing, very malignant, very vascular and to show early and widespread metastasis.

Particular problems of managing children include those of psychology (reassurance, establishing rapport, explanation), immobilisation (very young children may need to be sedated or even anaesthetised for certain investigations and therapy), infection (simple infections like measles, mumps and chickenpox can be fatal in the immunosuppressed child), metabolic upset (dangerous dehydration can occur very rapidly) and family contacts (these need to be maintained even though the child must be treated in a specialised centre).

The types and proportion of tumours seen in children are shown in Table 12.1. Haemopoietic tumours form the largest group of childhood malignancies, particularly acute lymphatic leukaemia. The management of malignant lymphoma is basically as in the adult patients (see Chapter 11). Histiocytosis X, if indeed it is a neoplasm, may be the most underdiagnosed of childhood tumours.

Neural tumours are the commonest of the solid tumours. In the central nervous system the majority of childhood tumours tend to be infratentorial, whereas in the adult most are supratentorial. The group includes astrocytomas—usually cerebellar, medulloblastoma, ependymoma and other gliomas. Surgery is usually the treatment of choice, often followed by central nervous system (CNS) irradiation. The overall survival is about 50% at 5 years but residual CNS defects are not uncommon. A full discussion of CNS tumours is given in Chapter 13. Neuroblastoma and retinoblastoma are discussed below. Sarcomas and other tumours are discussed in their relevant chapters.

Childhood leukaemia

This is most frequently of the acute form and of the lymphoblastic type. Chronic and acute myeloid leukaemia account for less than 5% of childhood leukaemias.

Table 12.1. Childhood tumours (commoner neoplasms within each group are italicised).

HAEMOPOIETIC	
Leukaemia, lymphoma, 'histiocytosis X'	40%
NEURAL	
Astrocytoma, medulloblastoma, retinoblastoma, other gliomas	25%
SARCOMA	
Osteogenic sarcoma, rhabdomyosarcoma, Ewing's sarcoma,	10%
KIDNEY	
Wilms' tumour	10%
OTHERS	
Adrenal, gonadal, hepatoblastoma	15%

Acute lymphoblastic leukaemia

Acute lymphoblastic leukaemia is rare at birth but the incidence increases sharply to a peak at about 4 years of age. The aetiology is unknown though environmental (irradiation, chemicals), viral (animal experiments, clustering of cases) and genetic (twin studies, associated genetic diseases, chromosomal studies) factors have all been implicated.

Clinical presentation

The presentation is by the effects of bone marrow or other tissue infiltration. The former may cause anaemia, thrombocytopenia with purpura and haemorrhagic diathesis, and neutropenia with increased risk of infection particularly of the throat. Other tissues commonly involved include lymph nodes, liver and spleen, all of which can be enlarged. In addition the child may be lethargic, pale or feverish and may have lost weight. Joint, bone and abdominal pain are sometimes seen. One variant of lymphatic leukaemia is the so-called Sternberg type where the initial presentation is of a large mediastinal mass; leukaemic T cells are subsequently found.

Differential diagnosis

The differential diagnosis includes infectious mononucleosis, various juvenile collagen–vascular disorders (rheumatic fever, rheumatoid arthritis, systemic lupus erythematosus) and other childhood malignancies.

The diagnosis is not normally difficult because leukaemic cells can be found in the peripheral blood examination. Occasionally, however, the white blood call count is normal and only a few abnormal cells can be seen, the so-called 'aleukaemic' leukaemia. Leukaemia must always be confirmed by a bone marrow examination with appropriate cytology and immunological typing of the leukaemic lymphocyte population involved. The use of immunological markers has identified several types of ALL. Three-quarters of cases are of the so-called 'common' type (recognised by the presence of the CALL antigen); less common are 'T' ALL and 'null' ALL. 'B' ALL is rare but almost uniformly lethal.

Probable prognosis

The probable prognosis of the patient may be assessed by a combination of clinical and laboratory indices (Table 12.2). The prognosis is better with girls, aged 2–8 years, with no significant organomegaly, with white cell count of less than $20 \times 10^9/1$ and platelets of more than $100 \times 10^9/1$, where small darkly stained lymphoblasts are found and with certain immunological types (e.g. 'C' ALL, 'null' ALL). Many of these factors are, of course, interrelated.

Treatment

The treatment of acute lymphoblastic leukaemia has seen major advances over the past 20 years. The first principle of management is to reduce the population of malignant cells to as near zero as possible by intensive chemotherapy. Remission is induced by a combination of cytotoxic agents (e.g. prednisolone, vincristine, and asparaginase). Once remission is induced

Table 12.2. Prognostic factors in acute lymphatic leukaemia.

1 Age
2 Sex
3 Organomegaly
4 Initial white cell count
5 Initial platelet count
6 Size of lymphoblast
7 Immunological type of lymphoblast

consolidation and maintenance treatment with drugs such as 6-mercapto-purine, methotroxate, cyclophosphamide is continued for up to 2 years or more.

It was realised very soon after the initial excellent responses to combination chemotherapy that certain pharmacological 'sanctuary' areas were commonly the sites of relapse. The central nervous system (particularly the meninges) was the most important and this is now routinely treated pro-phylatically by cranial irradiation and intrathecal cytotoxic chemotherapy, usually with methotrexate. It is now also realised that 10% of boys will develop testicular disease, posing the controversial question of prophylactic testicular irradiation.

In cases of marrow relapse the initial induction regimen may again be effective; other drugs in combination (e.g. doxorubicin, daunorubicin, cytosine arabinoside, nitrosoureas) may be used in non-responsive cases or further relapses. Bone marrow transplantation, where possible, is another alternative.

One of the biggest trials in leukaemia is the Medical Research Council United Kingdom Acute Lymphatic Leukaemia (UKALL) trial; several protocols have been tried and improved.

Supportive treatment is of vital importance particularly in the induction phase of treatment. Erythrocyte, platelet or leucocyte transfusion may be needed; infections must be treated early and energetically where possible, and uric acid nephropathy, from massive cell breakdown, must be avoided by appropriate use of allopurinol.

Results

The prognosis of acute lymphatic leukaemia has improved from its being an invariably fatal disease with most patients dying within a year of presentation to being a potentially curable disease; the overall cure rate is now 60% or more. Important prognostic factors have already been mentioned (Table 12.2).

Neuroblastoma

This is one of the commonest solid tumours of childhood with approximately the same incidence as nephroblastoma. Most occur below the age of 5 years, with half in the first 2 years of life. The tumour may be present at birth. It arises from sympathetic nervous tissue, particularly in the adrenal medulla, but also in the neck, mediastinum and pelvis. The tumour, histologically characterised by densely staining cells in neurofibrillar tissue and the presence of rosettes, invades locally, produces lymph node metastases, and disseminates via the bloodstream to the bones and liver.

Clinical presentation

Presenting symptoms may be related to the primary tumour mass, for example distended abdomen, or to metastases. Periorbital deposits are classical.

Intravenous pyelography is helpful in distinguishing the tumour from Wilms' tumour. Neuroblastomas produce catecholamines, and breakdown products (such as vanillyl-mandelic acid) can be measured in the urine, thus providing a useful diagnostic test and a means of monitoring tumour activity after treatment.

Management

Management includes surgery, radiotherapy and cytotoxic chemotherapy. Many tumours are too advanced for radical surgery, but partial removal can be helpful by reducing tumour bulk. Radiotherapy must cover a wide volume including the kidney on the side of the tumour; the opposite kidney is shielded in the latter part of treatment, otherwise permanent damage results. One regimen of chemotherapy is a combination of cyclical vincristine, cyclophosphamide and adriamycin for 4 months, followed by vincristine and cyclophosphamide only in cycles over at least 1 year. An alternative second-line agent is dacarbazine (DTIC).

Radical treatment uses all three modalities. Local radiotherapy to metastases can be of great palliative value.

Neuroblastomas undergo spontaneous regression or differentiation into benign ganglioneuromas in about 8% of cases.

Results

Results of treatment depend upon the stage of the disease and upon the age of the patient. The overall survival is about 40%; for truly localised disease it is above 80%. Below the age of 1 year 75% survive at least 2 years; above this age the figure is only about 20%. It has been suggested that immunological factors play a part in the better survival of the very young.

Nephroblastoma (Wilms' tumour)

Clinical presentation

The presentation of this tumour is most commonly as an intra-abdominal tumour arising from the renal cortex in a young child. There may also be haematuria, weight loss, anaemia and hypertension. Metastasis occurs via lymphatics and blood stream; the renal capsule may be breached. Bilateral tumours are found in about 5% of cases.

Aetiology

The aetiology is unknown but it may be associated with various congenital malformations (e.g. aniridia, hemihypertrophy, urinary tract anomalies).

Diagnosis

The diagnosis may be confirmed by plain X-ray (showing an opaque mass sometimes with peripheral calcification), intravenous pyelography, ultrasonography, CT scanning, arteriography and venography. A search for metastases, particularly in the lung, is vital.

Pathology

The pathological diagnosis is made from tissue removed at total nephrectomy; the predominant features are of embryonal round cells with an abundance of sarcoma-like tissue.

Treatment

Treatment is multimodal, after staging according to the investigative and surgical findings. Nephrectomy may be preceded by a few days of chemotherapy (e.g. with actinomycin D and/or vincristine) and is followed by total abdominal irradiation (using opposed fields with appropriate shielding of the contralateral kidney) and combination chemotherapy (actinomycin D, vincristine and sometimes doxorubicin) over an 18-month period.

Prognosis

The prognosis in this tumour, more than any other, demonstrates the effects of multimodal therapy. For patients with localised disease survivals of above 80% are now reported; even for widespread disease 60% survival is possible with chemotherapy.

Retinoblastoma

Retinoblastomas occur almost exclusively in children under the age of 5 and are bilateral in 30% of cases. Hereditary factors are undoubtedly important in the aetiology. The tumour usually metastasises late and often presents as a 'white pupil' or 'cat's eye' as the tumour reflects incident light. Visual disturbance and local pain may be present. Treatment is by enucleation in unilateral cases; in bilateral tumours the worst eye can be enucleated and the other treated with external irradiation. Advanced cases have been managed by combined radiotherapy and chemotherapy (e.g. vincristine and cyclophosphamide). Unilateral tumours have survival rates of over 80%; in bilateral and advanced cases survival falls to below 40%.

Histiocytosis X

Histiocytosis X is a disease of unknown aetiology characterised by the development of granulomatous lesions with abnormal proliferation of histiocytes; it is commonly believed to be a neoplastic disorder. It includes a variety of clinical syndromes including eosinophilic granuloma of bone, Hand–Schüller–Christian disease and reticuloendotheliosis (Letterer–Siwe disease), and the clinical course ranges from benign to highly malignant.

Letterer-Siwe disease represents an acute disseminated form of the disorder, seen most often in a child below 3 years of age. Hepatospleno-megaly, lymphadenopathy and skin, lung and bone infiltrations are found and the prognosis remains poor despite modern chemotherapy.

Hand–Schüller–Christian disease is a chronic disorder—usually the onset is in the age group 3–5 years and lesions are seen in bone and visceral tissues (skin, lung, lymph nodes and liver). The classical triad (cranial lesion, diabetes insipidus and exopthalmos) is seen only in a small proportion of cases. The course of the disease is slow and may become static; if death occurs it usually is from intracranial disease and infection.

Eosinophilic granuloma presents usually by bone lesions alone, in the age group 5–10 years; the prognosis is excellent and spontaneous regressions are seen.

In these disorders bone lesions may be treated with irradiation to relieve pain or to avert fractures. For widespread disease, particularly where the clinical deterioration is rapid, chemotherapy (e.g. vinca alkaloids, cyclophosphamide, methotrexate or prednisolone) can achieve sustained remissions.

Chapter 13
Tumours of the Central Nervous System

Primary tumours of the central nervous system account for about 2% of all tumours in man. The incidence is higher in white races than in negroes. There is no difference in sex incidence. They can arise at all ages, but the peak incidence of glial tumours is in childhood, when they are the commonest of solid tumours.

Causes

There are no known aetiological factors for these tumours. Trauma has been cited in some cases, but its role is not established.

Pathology

Malignant tumours of the central nervous system are unique in that they seldom metastasise outside their system of origin. Some have a strong tendency to spread within the cerebrospinal fluid pathways, for example medulloblastoma and ependymoblastoma. Occasionally medulloblastomas produce osteolytic bone metastases. Haemangioblastoma may be associated with histologically similar lesions in the retina and viscera.

Different areas in one tumour may show different grades of malignancy, especially in the astrocytoma group, and then the tumour is graded according to the least differentiated tissue present. The degree of malignancy also may increase with time; some tumours gradually become more anaplastic.

Tumours may be classified as follows:
1 Tumours of the glial (supportive) tissues—gliomas.
2 Tumours of the meninges and nerve sheaths.
3 Embryonal or vestigial tumours.
4 Mesenchymal tumours.
5 Other intracranial tumours.
6 Intracranial metastases.
7 Spinal cord tumours.

Gliomas

Gliomas account for about 50% of all primary brain tumours.

159

Astrocytomas

Astrocytomas account for about 75% of all gliomas. They are graded histologically from I to IV, based on decreasing degrees of differentiation. Astrocytomas may be cystic and haemorrhagic, particularly the less differentiated ones. Grade I tumours are slow growing and remain well demarcated. Typically they show collections of cells around blood vessels (rosette formation). The astrocytoma of the cerebellum which occurs in childhood is usually well differentiated and often has a good prognosis.

Grade IV astrocytoma, also known as glioblastoma, accounts for about half of all astrocytomas. It arises almost exclusively in the cerebral hemispheres or in the region of the basal ganglia. It is seldom circumscribed, usually infiltrates widely, may cross the midline via the corpus callosum, and may be multifocal in origin. It is a highly vascular tumour, and often produces oedema of the local normal brain tissues.

Ependymomas

Ependymomas arise in close proximity to the ventricular system of the brain, and may obstruct the cerebrospinal fluid pathways. Usually they are well differentiated and of low-grade malignancy, but obstructive effects may have fatal results. They occur both within the cranium and in the spinal canal (spinal cord and cauda equina), the distribution being approximately equal. They account for about 5% of all gliomas. A malignant form is described (ependymoblastoma).

Medulloblastomas

Medulloblastomas, forming about 10% of gliomas, are embryonal tumours. They are commonest in the first decade of life, but occasionally manifest their presence as late as the third decade. The commonest site is the floor of the fourth ventricle (cerebellar vermis).

Oligodendrogliomas

Oligodendrogliomas account for about 5% of all gliomas. Usually they have a rudimentary capsule; they may contain areas of calcification, demonstrable radiographically. Histologically they show a characteristic pseudo-epithelial arrangement of cells. Growth is slow, and tumours may attain a large size before causing symptoms.

Spongioblastoma

A tumour named spongioblastoma is described. It is rare. Usually it is of low-grade malignancy, is located in the brain stem or region of the optic chiasma, occurs in children, and is fairly radiosensitive despite its cytological features of low-grade malignancy.

Microglioma

The term microglioma is applied to the condition previously known as reticulum-cell sarcoma of the brain. It is a rare primary lymphoma of the brain. Its highest incidence is in the sixth and seventh decades of life; its sex incidence is equal.

It is responsive to radiation therapy initially, but long-term survival is rare. Cytotoxic chemotherapy may be of limited value in palliation, but few of the agents currently available penetrate brain tissue in significant amounts.

It should be noted that intracranial lymphoma may complicate generalised disease of this type, especially non-Hodgkin's lymphoma, and that the incidence of intracranial lymphoma is much higher in immunosuppressed patients than normal.

Tumours of the meninges and nerve sheaths

Tumours of the meninges and sheaths of intracranial nerves account for about 30% of primary central nervous system tumours.

Meningiomas

Meningiomas, which account for about two-thirds of the group, are commonest in the fifth decade of life. The majority are benign. Usually they are well defined (encapsulated) or spread as a sheet over the dura mater. Some are multilobular and calcification may be present within them. They may evoke a proliferation of adjacent bone or may produce local pressure absorption of bone; they seldom invade bone. Growth is usually slow, but an aggressive malignant form is described (meningiosarcoma). The commonest sites are the wings of the sphenoid and the tip of the petrous bone, the tuberculum sellae, the olfactory groove and the falx cerebri.

Acoustic neuroma and schwannomas

Tumours of the sheath of Schwann of the cranial nerves account for most of the remaining tumours in this group. They are termed schwannomas (neurilemmomas), or acoustic neuroma if on the auditory nerve which is the commonest site. Classically the latter tumour arises in the cerebellopontine angle; it produces unilateral deafness. These tumours are usually slow growing.

Rare intracranial tumours

Rarely intracranial fibromas, lipomas and melanomas are described; they are of little practical importance.

Embryonal tumours

Embryonal tumours, other than medulloblastoma previously mentioned, include craniopharyngioma and pinealoma.

Craniopharyngioma

Craniopharyngioma arises from residual cells of Rathke's pouch, a bud from the embryonal foregut which joins a downgrowth from the primitive midbrain to form the pituitary gland. The tumour typically consists mainly of a cyst cavity, the wall of which contains active cells sometimes concentrated in a knob of tumour. Growth of the tumour in children is more rapid than in adults, and obstruction of the foramen of Munroe may result. By virtue of its origin it lies in the region of the pituitary fossa; it may have pressure effects on the optic chiasma, and on the pituitary gland and hypothalamus thus giving rise to endocrine effects. Histologically, it is of low-grade malignancy.

Pinealoma

The term pinealoma is applied to a group of tumours which arise in the region of the pineal gland. They include teratomas, gliomas and meningiomas, and occasionally a seminoma-like tumour is described. Obstruction of the aqueduct of Silvius tends to occur early, with pronounced features of raised intracrancial pressure.

Mesenchymal tumours

Rare mesenchymal tumours include haemangiosarcoma and haemangioblastoma. The latter is usually benign and often is familial. Another type of vascular 'tumour' is the arteriovenous malformation. By definition it is a benign lesion, but haemorrhage from it can be considerable.

Other intracranial tumours

Other tumours include adenomas of the pituitary (see also Chapter 16), and the rare chromophobe carcinoma of the gland. Adenomas are classified according to the main cell type present; mixed tumours are not uncommon, but usually one cell type predominates.

Chromophobe adenoma, usually but not always hormonally inactive, accounts for about 80% of adenomas.

Eosinophil adenoma, so-called because the cells stain well with acidic dyes, produces giantism or acromegaly, depending upon the age of the person at the onset of activity.

Basophil adenoma or basophilism (diffuse hyperplasia), so-called because the cells stain well with basic dyes, produces Cushing's syndrome.

Chromophobe carcinoma shows the cytological features of malignancy, and has a tendency to invade locally.

Recently pituitary adenomas which secrete abnormally large amounts of prolactin have been described (prolactinomas). Usually they are small in size. Galactorrhoea may be a distressing symptom, amenorrhoea is usual, and infertility may be the presenting feature.

As a pituitary adenoma enlarges it produces pressure absorption of the bony walls of the fossa and stretching of the diaphragma sellae. The latter may be breached and the adenomatous mass extends upwards, producing pressure effects on the optic chiasma, and in some cases on the hypothalamus also.

Intracranial metastases

The commonest intracranial tumours are metastases. Primary carcinoma of the bronchus accounts for about 50% of these; other primary sites, approximately in descending order of incidence, include breast, gastrointestinal tract, kidney and skin (especially malignant melanoma).

Spinal cord tumours

Primary spinal cord tumours are not common; metastases account for the majority of malignant tumours in this site. They are divided into intramedullary and extramedullary groups. All the tumours included in the glioma group of intracranial lesions may arise in the spinal cord. Often they progress more slowly than their intracranial counterparts. Extramedullary tumours include haemangioma, neurofibroma, connective tissue sarcomas, meningioma and lymphoma.

Clinical features

The signs and symptoms of tumours of the central nervous system may be general or local.

General changes

General changes are related to an increase in the intracranial pressure. Obstruction to the flow of cerebrospinal fluid (CSF) or impairment of its reabsorption will result in an accumulation of fluid in the system with an increase in the CSF pressure and distension of the ventricles. This produces the classical picture of headache, vomiting and papilloedema, which may progress to impairment of mental function and reduced level of consciousness, and to coma and even to death. Papilloedema is associated with reduced visual acuity, and long-sustained papilloedema can result in optic atrophy.

A rise in the intracranial pressure can lead to impaction of the brain stem in the opening in the tentorium, or of the medulla in the foramen magnum, and either situation can result in rapid death, from depression of vital centres. False localising signs (e.g. sixth nerve paralysis due to stretching of the nerve on its long intracranial cause) also occur.

Sudden changes in the neurological state or level of consciousness may be due to haemorrhage into or around a tumour.

Local symptoms

Local symptoms and signs result from pressure upon, or destruction of, nerve cells and fibres, the particular features being related to the site of the tumour. Hemianopia classically results from optic chiasma compression by pituitary tumours; bitemporal hemianopia is usually quoted as the classical type, but other combinations of hemianopia or of quadrantic defects are not uncommon, depending upon the precise mechanism operative.

Paralyses of single or multiple cranial nerves may be demonstrable. For example, anosmia may be due to a meningioma in the olfactory groove, external ocular pareses may be due to a tumour adjacent to the cavernous sinus, and deafness may be due to an acoustic neuroma. Nystagmus and incoordination of the limbs typically occurs with cerebellar tumours. Damage to long tract fibres may produce unilateral pareses or disturbances of sensation. Tumours of the dominant temporal lobe may give speech defects. Tumours in the region of the cerebral motor cortex can produce fits of Jacksonian type; tumours in less well-defined motor areas may produce generalised epileptiform fits.

Incontinence or retention of urine and faeces may be related to intracranial or spinal cord tumours. Classically such disturbances result from damage to nerve fibres in the lumbar segments of the cord. Acute damage produces retention; more gradual changes tend to produce incontinence.

Spinal cord tumours may be localised accurately on their associated symptoms and signs. The upper limit of a zone of impaired sensation to pinprick is a precise indication of the spinal cord segment at the upper limit of a tumour. Changes in the limb tendon reflexes can also be related to changes at specific levels in the cord. Changes in the tone of the limb muscles is a less precise indication of the level of cord damage, but a spastic paraplegia indicates a lesion of the cord proper, whereas a flaccid paraplagia may be related to a tumour in the cauda equina.

Investigations

A full and detailed history and a meticulous clinical examination will usually indicate accurately the site of a tumour in the central nervous system and sometimes its probable nature. However, a decision about the best form of management requires very precise knowledge of the extent as well as the site of the lesion, and a firm histological diagnosis.

The simplest investigation is radiography of the skull with lateral, anteroposterior and basal views, or of the spinal column, as appropriate. Skull X-ray films may show evidence of raised intracranial pressure, more often demonstrable in children than in adults, displacement of the pineal gland if this is calcified, calcification within a tumour itself, new bone formation associated with a tumour, or bone destruction locally in the flat bones or in the pituitary fossal. Spinal X-ray films may show bone destruction in the vertebrae, sometimes associated with a paravertebral soft tissue mass.

Tomograms of localised areas taken in the anteroposterior or lateral planes may be useful, particularly in assessing the pituitary fossa and the petrous temporal bone.

The presence and extent of a tumour may be inferred from local vascular changes. Some tumours have abnormal circulations; others displace the normal vessels. An arteriovenous malformation will show gross vascular changes. Arteriography therefore plays an important role in assessment.

Contrast studies of the ventricular system of the brain or of the subarachnoid space of the spinal cord can also be helpful. The CSF in the ventricles can be replaced by air (air-encephalography) or by radio-opaque medium; the latter also can be introduced into the spinal subarachnoid space. Any displacement or irregularity of the cavities so outlined may be of diagnostic value.

Radioisotope scanning has proved a great value as a non-invasive technique in the investigation of intracranial tumours; it is of less value in respect of spinal tumours (see also Chapter 2).

In recent years, the development of computerised axial tomography (CT scanning) has revolutionised the location of intracranial tumours, and has also proved of some value in the demonstration of spinal cord tumours. In many cases, the appearance of a lesion on the film of a 'cut' of the brain will also suggest the histological nature of the tumour. Many tumours selectively take up contrast medium injected intravenously, thereby enhancing the radiological features. The radiation dose delivered to the patient in this investigation is not trivial, but carefully selected 'cuts' can be obtained with doses well within the acceptable limits. CT scanning is non-invasive, and as such has replaced ventriculography and arteriography to a large extent. There are situations, however, in which the latter two investigations still provide useful information not available from CT scanning (see also Chapter 2).

Ultrasound scanning has proved of limited value in the investigation of central nervous system tumours. The midline structures can be clearly depicted and any displacement shown. Attempts to define actual tumour masses within the skull have been disappointing.

Electroencephalography (EEG) has been used in the past to localise intracranial tumours, and is still of limited value.

Examination of the cerebrospinal fluid removed as a diagnostic procedure or at contrast radiography of the ventricular system and spinal subarachnoid space may yield information of value, for example the presence of tumour cells (occasionally) or an excess of protein if there is spinal obstruction above the site of puncture. It may indicate an alternative diagnosis.

More recently still, nuclear magnetic resonance (NMR) or magnetic resonance imaging (MRI) has been added to the investigational techniques available.

Management

The initial approach in management of intracranial tumours is usually surgery. This may be simple aspiration burr-hole biopsy, or craniotomy with open biopsy, partial removal of tumour or attempted total tumour excision. Either of the latter two procedures will reduce the bulk of the intracranial contents and achieve an internal decompression. If the intracranial pressure is raised due to obstruction in the ventricular system and substantial amounts of tumour cannot be removed it may be possible to insert a bypass tube from one lateral ventricle to the right atrium of the heart.

The value of an accurate histological diagnosis must be stressed. However, there are centrally located lesions for which it would be hazardous to attempt biopsy, and occasionally a tentative diagnosis must be made, based on the patient's age, history, and clinical and radiological features. The development of fine needle stereotactic biopsy techniques has made it possible to obtain tissue from almost any area within the skull, without unacceptable risks.

Complete surgical removal of intracranial tumours is seldom possible. The low-grade astrocytoma of cerebellum in childhood, and localised grade I astrocytoma of cerebrum in adults, are exceptions. Rarely postoperative radiotherapy is given if there is limited local residue.

Some other tumours are notoriously radioresistant; the best examples are poorly differentiated astrocytomas (grade III and IV). Others are very radiosensitive (e.g. medulloblastoma and ependymoblastoma), and although irradiation of the primary site and probable sites of dissemination of these tumours requires the treatment of large volumes, this is well tolerated at the dose levels necessary, and results are relatively good.

Pituitary adenoma tissue, especially that of chromophobe adenomas, is radiosensitive. However, initial surgery is essential if there is evidence of optic chiasma compression. The development of the transnasal transsphenoidal approach to the pituitary fossa has made removal of adenomas much safer; however complete clearance is virtually impossible, and postoperative irradiation is used. The sensitivity of eosinophil and basophil adenoma tissue is less than that of chromophobe tissue. Bromocriptine has proved of value in reducing elevated serum levels of growth hormone and of prolactin in some cases of eosinophil and prolactin adenomas.

Meningiomas are radioresistant, and radiotherapy plays no part in their management. The same is true in general of acoustic neuromas, except that a technique for high-dose high-intensity single exposure treatments to very localised volumes has been developed in Sweden, and has yielded encouraging results.

Craniopharyngiomas may respond to full-dose irradiation. The place of radiotherapy in the management of pinealomas depends upon the histological type of tumour; non-glial tumours may show some response. Arteriovenous malformations not amenable to surgery may be irradiated; responses are slow, and may not be fully developed for 18 months or 2 years.

Spinal cord tumours may require urgent treatment. Developing paraparesis or recently established paraplegia calls for immediate laminectomy to decompress the cord. It may be possible to make a tentative diagnosis before operation; often the histological nature of the tumour is known only after microscopic examination of removed tissue. The technical difficulty

of achieving total removal of cord tumours makes postoperative radiotherapy necessary in many cases. Urinary and faecal retention or incontinence may complicate the clinical situation, and call for appropriate
management.

The treatment of metastases in the brain is of limited value. In general,
radiotherapy is indicated only if the primary tumour has proved sensitive
(e.g. undifferentiated small cell carcinoma of bronchus). If the primary
tumour is in the thyroid and has shown radioiodine uptake, treatment
using this isotope may be of value. If the primary tumour is in the breast
and is hormone dependent this form of treatment is indicated. Occasionally,
an apparently solitary slow-growing metastasis in an accessible site is
removed surgically.

The physical effects of spinal cord metastases and the commonly associated local pain require treatment by radiation in most cases. This may prevent the development of paraplegia, and if cord damage is not already extensive or of long duration may result in some neurological recovery.

Normal brain tissue is less tolerant of radiation damage than many other
normal tissues, this being especially true of the hypothalamus and brain
stem; also, brain tissue in children is less tolerant than in adults.

Radiotherapy techniques

In the rare cases in which radiotherapy is given after subtotal removal of a
grade I or II astrocytoma, ependymoma or oligodendroglioma, small field
high-dose treatment is used. The results from radiotherapy alone for grade
III and IV astrocytomas are so poor that such treatment is not usually
indicated.

Treatment of medulloblastomas and ependymoblastomas requires the irradiation of the whole of the cerebrospinal axis, down to the lower border
of the second sacral vertebra (that is, to cover the whole of the CSF
pathway).

Pituitary adenomas are treated using small fields, and a cellulose acetate
shell for accurate beam direction. Basophil adenomas may require higher
doses than the chromophobe variety, and for eosinophil adenomas the very
high local doses from implanted yttrium-90 pellets are usually recommended. Proton beams have also been used.

Craniopharyngiomas are treated by a similar external radiation technique. Pinealomas regarded as localised are treated similarly; so also are
arteriovenous malformations.

Primary spinal cord tumours may be irradiated, after preliminary
surgical decompression, if there is obvious or suspected residue. Radiotherapy as palliation also has a place.

Radiotherapy in the palliation of intracranial metastases usually requires whole brain irradiation. An alternative to radiotherapy is single agent cytotoxic chemotherapy in the form of oral CCNU.

Radiotherapy will produce epilation; at the highest dose levels this will be permanent, otherwise hair regrowth can be expected 2 or 3 months after treatment. Radiation skin reaction in the scalp is usually mild but may be brisker in the postauricular areas.

The problems of raised intracranial pressure have been greatly alleviated by the use of dexamethasone, which in favourable cases will control the pressure until the cause can be treated. In other cases it may be of temporary palliative value.

Prognosis

Surgical treatment of grade I and II astrocytomas yields 5-year survival rates of about 25%; it has been reported that this can be increased to about 50% by the addition of radiotherapy. The infratentorial astrocytoma of childhood shows better results—75% at 5 years from surgery alone. Grade III and IV astrocytomas show survivals of less than 5% at 1 year.

Treatment of medulloblastomas results in 5-year survival figures of about 45%. It is claimed that about 30% of patients are cured.

Figures quoted for chromophobe adenomas of the pituitary are 30% recurrence-free at 4 years from surgery alone, 75% from radiotherapy alone, and 93% for combined surgery and radiotherapy. The results for eosinophil and basophil adenomas are less impressive. Treatment of eosinophil adenomas may improve symptoms, but does not increase life expectancy.

Treatment of craniopharyngioma results in long-term survival in many cases, and long-term control of pinealomas can often be achieved.

Chapter 14
Tumours of Bone and
Soft Tissue

The mesenchymal layer of the embryo develops into connective tissue, bone, muscle, fat, blood vessels and blood cells and lymph nodes. Malignancies arising in these tissues are termed sarcomas, endotheliomas, leukaemias and lymphomas, depending upon the tissue affected.

Despite the common developmental origin of this large group of malignancies, they show two widely different levels of sensitivity to irradiation, and can thereby be divided into two separate groups:

1 Very sensitive tumours—for example, the lymphoreticular malignancies.

2 Very resistant tumours—for example, the connective tissue sarcomas.

Only rarely are examples found in either group which do not follow the pattern of the two extremes of radiation response.

It has been suggested that this difference may be related to the fact that early in the development of the embryo, some elements of the mesenchyme differentiate into tissues with highly specialised functions, such as bone and muscle, whereas others persist throughout life in a relatively undifferentiated state for the purpose of defence, tissue repair and blood formation. This difference fits well with the expected degree of radiosensitivity or radioresistance, the less differentiated tissues being sensitive and the well differentiated tissues being resistant.

The lymphomas and leukaemias are considered in Chapter 11. The sarcomas of bone, muscle and connective tissue can be classified as follows:

1 Osteosarcoma.
2 Chondrosarcoma.
3 Osteoclastoma.
4 Ewing's sarcoma.
5 Chordoma.
6 Synoviosarcoma.
7 Fibrosarcoma.
8 Myosarcoma,
  a leiomyosarcoma,
  b rhabdomyosarcoma.
9 Liposarcoma.
10 Neurosarcoma.
11 Malignant fibrohistiocytoma.

Osteosarcoma

Osteosarcoma is the commonest of the primary malignant tumours of bone, accounting for about 40%.

Incidence

Its highest incidence is in the second decade of life, when about 70% arise. Tumours of this type in later life usually represent malignant change in an area of Paget's disease of bone, or malignant change in a pre-existing osteoclastoma, or are secondary to the local effects of deposits of radioactive elements in the bone, for example radium and strontium.

Osteosarcoma is commoner in males than in females in the ratio 2 : 1.

Sites

The commonest sites are the lower end of the femur (about 40%), the upper end of the tibia (20%), the upper end of the humerus (10%) and the pelvic bones (10%). Childhood lesions develop most commonly in the metaphyses of long bones.

Symptoms

Pain is the commonest symptom; later there is local swelling. There may be venous congestion and local heat. The lesion may present as a pathological fracture. Blood borne metastases occur early, usually to the lungs, but occasionally to other bones also.

Radiography

Radiographs show osteolysis, osteosclerosis or both. There may be evidence of new bone formation. Some tumours show the so-called sun-ray appearance due to radiating spicules of bone, and there may be a Codman's triangle of periostial new bone at the limits of the bony changes. The actual extent of the tumour in the bone marrow cavity may be much greater than would be judged from the radiological changes.

Treatment

Treatment is by amputation if technically possible. This may be done as the primary procedure, or high-dose radiation therapy may be given and this followed 6–9 months later by amputation if the lungs remain radiologically free of metastases. The latter regimen was introduced because of the high incidence of lung metastases evident soon after amputation in many cases, and it was intended to avoid mutilating surgery to a young adult who was to succumb shortly thereafter to distant metastases.

If the primary tumour is not in a limb, or if amputation is refused, the whole of the affected bone and demonstrable soft tissue involvement with a wide bony margin can be irradiated to a high dose, using supervoltage radiation.

Nowadays, cytotoxic chemotherapy is added to the treatment regimen, in an attempt to deal with small distant metastases, which inevitably must be present in many cases at the time of operation. The agents used are vincristine and methotrexate, with or without doxorubicin. The methotrexate is given in high doses, and its continued effects neutralised after an interval by administration of an antagonist, folinic acid (see Chapter 4).

Combined treatments increase the disease-free interval after initial treatment, but it is not clear whether overall survival is increased. Quoted figures are of 50% in remission at 1 year, and 40% alive at 2 years.

Chondrosarcoma

Chondrosarcoma is a malignant tumour of cartilage cells. It may arise as malignant change in a previously benign osteochondroma (1%), or in a focus of multiple enchondroma (about 20%); less commonly it arises as malignant changes in a pure chondroma. It can arise *de novo* as a malignant tumour.

It is less common than osteosarcoma, accounting for about 10% of primary malignant bone tumours. It shows no difference in sex incidence.

Incidence, sites and symptoms

Its highest incidence is in the age range 10–25 years. The commonest sites are the lower end of the femur and the upper ends of the tibia and humerus.

Pain is the commonest symptom, with later local swelling, but the local changes may develop insidiously.

Radiography

Radiographically there is irregular destruction of the bone, with some periostial new bone formation and often with a Codman's triangle.

Local extent is again greater than that indicated radiographically. Pulmonary metastases are common, but usually at a much later stage of the disease than in osteosarcoma.

Treatment

Treatment is surgical; these tumours are very radioresistant, though sometimes local palliative radiotherapy can reduce swelling and ease pain. Cytotoxic chemotherapy is of very limited value.

Overall 5-year survival figures of about 35% are quoted.

Osteoclastoma

Osteoclastoma, also known as giant cell tumour of bone, is of uncertain origin, but is usually classified as a bone tumour. It is composed of osteo-clast-like cells. Usually it is benign; however, about 15% become malignant or are malignant from the outset.

It is not common, accounting for about 5% of primary malignant bone tumours. Most arise in early adult life (20–40 years of age). It is a little commoner in males than in females.

Sites

The commonest sites are the ends of the long bones, with the lower end of the femur and the upper end of the tibia accounting for about half the cases, and the upper end of the femur, the lower end of the radius and the upper end of the humerus accounting for about a quarter of cases.

Almost always these tumours are solitary with either local pain or, not uncommonly, a pathological fracture as the presenting features. There may be palpable local 'egg-shell crackling' demonstrable, due to thin layers of expanded bone around the tumour. Radiologically, a 'soap-bubble' appearance due to persisting bone trabeculae within the tumour area is characteristic.

Treatment

Lesions amenable to surgical excision are best treated by this method, with bone grafting if necessary. Those less accessible to excision may be curetted, and the cavity swabbed with phenol solution and packed with bone chips. Otherwise, radiotherapy is indicated, although it has been suggested that this may be a factor in the later development of malignant change in some tumours.

Ewing's sarcoma

Ewing's sarcoma is a small-cell sarcoma of bone, which may also be classified as a lymphoreticular malignancy. It occurs in childhood and early adult life (5–20 years of age). It accounts for about 2% of childhood malignancies. It is commoner in males than in females.

Sites

The commonest sites are the femur, humerus, tibia, pelvis and ribs. It arises within, and widely infiltrates, the marrow cavity. It has a marked tendency to metastasise early, particularly to the lungs, other bones and the brain.

Symptoms

It can mimic an infective condition by producing local redness, swelling and heat, fever, raised peripheral white blood cell count and raised ESR. Biopsy confirmation of the diagnosis is therefore essential.

Treatment

Surgery is usually confined to biopsy only, although amputation for a primary tumour of a limb has been advocated because of the impairment of bone growth in young patients resulting from radiotherapy and cytotoxic chemotherapy. Nevertheless, established treatment is to irradiate the whole of the affected bone. This is followed by combination chemotherapy; one popular regimen consists of cyclophosphamide, vincristine and doxorubicin every 2 weeks for six treatments, followed by cyclophosphamide, vincristine and actinomycin-D monthly to 2 years.

Currently quoted results are 50% alive and well at 2 years.

Chordoma

Chordoma is a tumour arising in remnants of the notocord of the embryo. It is sited in the spheno-occipital area in about 40% of cases, and in the sacrococcygeal area in about 45% of cases; the remaining 15% arise along the intervening spinal column.

Treatment

It is of limited radiosensitivity, and treatment should be by surgical excision if possible. As complete excision is often not possible because of site, radiotherapy may be indicated, but is seldom of other than palliative value. Nevertheless, pain relief and growth restraint may be achieved.

Synoviosarcoma

Synoviosarcoma is a rare tumour which originates in the synovial membrane of joints. Tumours similar to synoviosarcoma sometimes arise in other endothelial tissues such as the pleura, peritoneum and the meninges of the brain.

Synoviosarcomas tend to be slow growing initially, but later the rate of growth may accelerate. Occasionally, they show some response to irradiation, being a little less resistant than osteosarcomas and chondrosarcomas. However, if radical surgical excision is possible it is the treatment of choice.

Fibrosarcoma

Fibrosarcoma may arise primarily in bone endosteal connective tissue or in connective tissues elsewhere in the body. Primary fibrosarcoma may show a wide spectrum of malignancy. It is not common, representing about 7% of all primary malignant bone tumours, and is uncommon below the age of 30 years.

Sites

The commonest sites are the femur and the tibia, and pathological fracture through the tumour site can occur.

Treatment

Treatment is by radical surgical excision if possible, with a wide margin for anaplastic tumours and a smaller margin for well-differentiated ones. It may be a little more radiosensitive than osteosarcoma and chondrosarcoma, and radiotherapy may be of some value for localised tumours not amenable to excision. Cytotoxic chemotherapy is of very limited value.

The management of soft tissue fibrosarcomas is along similar lines to that of bone fibrosarcomas.

Overall 5-year survival is about 40%.

Myosarcoma

Myosarcoma is a malignant tumour of muscle, and can be subdivided into leiomyosarcoma (arising from smooth muscle) and rhabdomyosarcoma (arising from striated muscle). Smooth muscle is found mainly in the gut wall and in the myometrium, and malignant change in a uterine fibroid is one form of leiomyosarcoma.

Rhabdomyosarcomas can be subdivided into embryonal, botryoid (resembling a bunch of grapes), alveolar and pleomorphic types. The embryonal variety is the most common type and usually arises in the head and neck region or in relation to the genitalia in childhood; it may be of botryoid form especially in the female genitourinary tract. The alveolar variety usually arises in the limbs. The pleomorphic type is the classical one of adults. Local infiltration is common and lymphatic and haematogenous spread can occur early.

Treatment

In general, myosarcomas are very radioresistant, and the only potentially curative treatment is radical surgical excision. However, local radiotherapy may be of palliative value.

The rhabdomyosarcoma of childhood may respond well to combined surgery, radiotherapy and cytotoxic chemotherapy. The surgery may be an attempt at excision or merely a biopsy, depending on the site and extent of the tumour. Radiotherapy doses must be fairly high. One regimen of chemotherapy combines vincristine, actinomycin-D and cyclophosphamide given in a single session, weekly for 6 weeks, followed by fortnightly injections for 1 year.

Five-year survival figures of about 60% are being claimed.

Liposarcoma

Liposarcoma is a rare tumour, perhaps surprisingly so in view of the high incidence of its benign counterpart—simple lipoma.

Little can be said about its management except that the only chance of cure lies in radical surgical excision; radiotherapy and chemotherapy are ineffective.

Neurosarcoma

Neurosarcoma also is rare, again surprisingly so, as its benign counterpart (neurofibroma) is not uncommon.

Yet again, it is resistant to radiation therapy, and was regarded as resistant to chemotherapy until recently. Now responses are claimed for a combination of doxorubicin and dacarbazine (DTIC). These responses have not been complete or permanent, but indicate that there is some hope for palliation in these tumours, previously regarded as entirely resistant. Another recently reported regimen adds vincristine and cyclophosphamide to doxorubicin and dacarbazine.

These comments on the response of neurosarcomas to chemotherapy can now be applied to other malignant tumours of mesenchymal origin. They were regarded as generally resistant, but newer agents and newer combinations are yielding better results, especially when used to supplement radical surgical excision.

Malignant fibrohistiocytoma

The term malignant fibrohistiocytoma covers a group of tumours having a common origin from tissue histiocytes. In the past, tumours of this type have been diagnosed as pleomorphic rhabdomyosarcoma or undifferentiated fibrosarcoma. These lesions usually arise in the deeper connective tissues of the body. They may reach a large size yet remain fairly well defined, and wide surgical excision may be curative. The more aggressive tumours infiltrate widely and metastasise. They show limited radiosensitivity; cytotoxic chemotherapy may be of limited value in palliation.

Chapter 15
Skin Cancer

Skin cancer is one of the commonest human malignancies. Basal cell carcinoma accounts for over half, and squamous cell carcinoma for over a quarter, of all skin cancer. The remaining proportion is made up of melanoma, secondary skin metastases, lymphoma and various other uncommon lesions.

Basal cell carcinoma

Basal cell carcinoma (rodent ulcer) occurs with greater incidence in white races with excessive sunlight exposure, as for example in Australia. It may occur in a dominantly inherited condition, the basal cell naevus syndrome. About three-quarters of basal cell carcinomas arise in the head and neck region, characteristically as an ulcerated nodule. Clinically there may be some difficulty in distinguishing the lesion from kerato-acanthoma, which typically has a central core of keratin. The remainder of basal cell carcinomas occur elsewhere on the body; occasional difficulty is experienced in distinguishing these from solar keratoses, though the latter do not have the typical raised rolled edges of the rodent ulcer.

Metastases are very rare from basal cell carcinoma; if death occurs it is usually from infiltration of vital structures, particularly the brain where infection is often the cause of death.

Treatment

Treatment is curative in the great majority (over 90%) of cases and this can be by surgical excision (if easily accessible) or by local radiotherapy. Other less favoured methods of treatment include electrocautery, cryosurgery and topical cytotoxic chemotherapy (e.g. fluorouracil ointment). In general the patient can receive out-patient treatment unless very elderly or otherwise infirm. Great care must be taken to ensure a good cosmetic result in facial lesions.

Recurrent lesions can frequently be cured by the form of treatment alternative to that first used.

Squamous cell carcinoma

Squamous cell carcinoma (Marjolin's ulcer) occurs with increased frequency in non-pigmented skin, excessive sunlight exposure, chemical carcinogenesis (e.g. with coal tar products), and with chronic irritation. A recessively inherited skin condition, xeroderma pigmentosum, is associated with development of squamous cell carcinoma. Over half of the lesions occur in the head and neck region and about a quarter on the arms and hands.

Bowen's disease, usually manifested as brownish-red crusted or eroded skin plaques, is a form of intraepidermal carcinoma which may become invasive after a period of months or years. It is also acknowledged to be a herald marker of internal malignancy, particularly bronchial carcinoma.

Differential diagnosis of squamous carcinoma from basal cell carcinoma and from solar keratosis may be difficult; the squamous lesion is frequently nodular and ulcerated, but may be flat and keratotic. Histological confirmation is required; at the same time an idea of the degree of differentiation and local invasion can be obtained.

Treatment

Localised lesions which are well differentiated histologically and forming keratin pearls are curable in the majority (greater than 90%) of cases by adequate excisional surgery, though results with radiotherapy are also excellent. Larger poorly differentiated lesions may infiltrate extensively and may metastasise by lymphatic and vascular invasion. Surgery may still be appropriate but radiotherapy is particularly useful in this group. Disseminated disease occasionally responds to combination cytotoxic chemotherapy.

Malignant melanoma

Malignant melanoma, a tumour which strikes fear into the heart of even the most experienced of oncologists, is in fact an uncommon tumour, accounting for less than 1% of total cancers. In the skin it is seen with most frequency, as with basal cell and squamous cell lesions, in fair-skinned races exposed to excessive sunlight, as for example in Australia.

Pathology

Pathologically skin melanoma is divided into three types:
1 Lentigo maligna, a flat dark brown lesion occurring classically on the head and neck region of the older patient.

2 Superficial spreading melanoma, flat and extending, usually nearly black in colour.

3 Nodular melanoma, sometimes ulcerated and usually dark brown.

Occasionally a melanoma may not be pigmented (amelanotic melanoma). Survival is best with lentigo maligna and worst with nodular melanoma; superficial spreading melanoma comes between these two. Prognosis also depends on the level of invasion in the skin of the melanoma, the deeper the spread the worse the prognosis.

Differential diagnosis

Malignant melanoma developing in a pigmented mole is uncommon, but may occur more frequently in naevi on the palms and soles. A difficult differential diagnostic problem is of course between the mole and the malignant melanoma; in general, lesions with changing size or pigmentation, ulceration or bleeding, should be excised and examined histologically.

Treatment

Treatment of the primary melanoma must be by surgery with wide excision of surrounding skin. Prophylactic regional lymph node dissection has been advocated for tumours with clinically or histologically aggressive features. If there is no evidence of metastasis survival figures are excellent (greater than 90% at 5 years). Once metastasis has occurred however the outlook is much worse with 5-year survival of less than 10%. Spread occurs via superficial lymphatics, giving satellite lesions, via deep lymphatics to regional lymph nodes and via the blood stream most often to lung, liver and brain. Block dissection of regional nodes or regional arterial perfusion of cytotoxics is occasionally effective. In general radiotherapy, chemotherapy and immunotherapy have little to offer except in palliation.

Malignant lymphoma

Malignant lymphoma occurs occasionally as true cutaneous deposits in both Hodgkin's disease and non-Hodgkin's lymphoma. Specific T cell skin lymphomas are also seen (see Chapter 11). The Sézary syndrome, of erythroderma with lymphocytic skin infiltration and abnormal blood lymphocytes, and mycosis fungoides, a cutaneous lymphoma characteristically progressing from non-specific 'premycotic' erythroderma to a stage of indurated neoplastic plaques, can both develop into systemic lymphoreticular malignancies. Treatment of isolated lymphoma deposits by radiotherapy gives excellent results; the treatment of widespread lymphoma is much less satisfactory. Superficial whole body irradiation, systemic chemotherapy and more recently the use of psoralen and ultraviolet light (PUVA) therapy can be helpful in many patients.

Metastatic skin tumours

Metastatic skin tumours, particularly from breast, lung or gastrointestinal tract, are not usually difficult to diagnose. Treatment is palliative and most often by irradiation, particularly when the lesion is ulcerated or painful.

Other rare tumours

Other rare tumours can arise from structures in the dermis, for example from blood vessels, fibrous tissue and sweat glands. Treatment of these is primarily by excisional surgery.

Kaposi's sarcoma

Kaposi's sarcoma probably arises from the skin blood vessels and has a classical histological appearance. Though clinically often a slowly progressive multifocal skin disease, widespread visceral changes occur eventually in the majority of patients. Treatment of the skin lesion is by surgery or radiotherapy; disseminated disease occasionally responds to chemotherapy. There is an increased incidence of second cancer (particularly of the reticuloendothelial system) in patients with Kaposi's sarcoma. This neoplasm is a common feature in the 'aquired immunodeficiency syndrome' (see page 10); its behaviour is much more aggressive in this group.

Chapter 16
Paraneoplastic (Non-Metastatic) and Hormonal Syndromes Associated with Tumours

Cancers manifest their presence in three ways, firstly by the presence of the primary tumour and its local spread, secondly by metastasis to secondary sites, and thirdly by their remote, non-metastic, effects on various tissues. These remote effects often form specific clinical syndromes which may be markers of the underlying cancer. They occur in more than 15% of patients; their pathogenesis is, however, poorly understood except perhaps in the case of the endocrine syndromes. Metabolic, toxic, immunological and endocrine factors have all been suggested in the pathogenesis of the various general, dermatological, neurological and haematological syndromes. The important remote effects and the types of tumour most likely to be responsible are tabulated (Table 16.1).

Hormonal disturbances associated with oversecretion by tumours (apudomas) of substances appropriate to the tumour's tissue of origin are discussed in this chapter because of their relevance to the understanding of the 'paraneoplastic' endocrinopathies.

Table 16.1. Non-metastatic effects of cancers.

Effect	Tumour
GENERAL	
Anorexia, cachexia, malaise	
Pyrexia	Advanced malignancy
Metabolic	
Fever	
ENDOCRINE	
Adrenocortical hyperplasia	Oat cell bronchogenic carcinoma
Hypercalcaemia	Breast carcinoma, myeloma
Inappropriate antidiuresis	Oat cell bronchogenic carcinoma
Hypoglycaemia	Retroperitoneal sarcoma
Hyperthyroidism	Choriocarcinoma
Precocious puberty	Hepatoblastoma
Gynaecomastia/HPOA	Bronchogenic carcinoma
Apudomas	Multiple

DERMATOLOGICAL

Non-specific
  infective
  pruritus   }   Any malignancy, particularly
  ichthyosis   lymphomas
  haemorrhage
Specific
  acanthosis nigricans   Adenocarcinoma
  exfoliative erythroderma   Malignant lymphoma
  dermatomyositis   Lung, GI tract, breast
  tylosis   Oesophagus
  erythema gyratum repens   Lung, breast
  malignant down   Bladder, lung

NEUROLOGICAL

Brain and spinal cord
  cerebellar degeneration
  encephalomyelitis   }   Usually lung
  dementia
  motor neurone disease
Nerves
  various neuropathies   Any malignancy
Muscles
  myopathy   Any malignancy
  myasthenia   Lung
  polymyositis   GI tract, lung

HAEMATOLOGICAL

Anaemia   Advanced malignancy
Erythrocytosis   Kidney
White cell abnormality
  leucocytosis   }   Advanced malignancy
  leucopenia
Platelet abnormality
  thrombocytosis   }   Advanced malignancy
  thrombocytopenia
Hypercoagulability   Pancreas, lung, GI tract
Hyperviscosity   Myeloma, macroglobulinaemia
Haemorrhage   Any advanced malignancy
Immunosuppression   Lymphoma, leukaemia,
                               advanced carcinoma

General effects

The patient with cancer, particularly when this is widespread, feels generally ill, loses his or her appetite (anorexia) and shows a disproportionate weight loss (cachexia). Various abnormalities of carbohydrate, protein and lipid metabolism are thought to underly these symptoms. The dietary intake of vital food substances is reduced and mechanical (e.g. tumour pressure), and non-specific (e.g. the effects of drugs) factors may give rise to abnormalities of bowel motility and food processing, resulting in varying degrees of malabsorption. Muscle protein catabolism occurs in the ill, immobile patient and a negative protein balance ensues. Carbohydrate and lipid stores are also utilised inappropriately to provide the excess of energy needed in this stress situation.

In addition there is often, in association with anaemia and infection, impaired cellular respiration. The net result which may be compounded by vitamin and vital element deficiency and electrolyte/fluid disorders results in a disproportionate weight loss or cachexia, often the forerunner of death.

Electrolyte disturbances

Electrolyte disturbances are common in the patient with cancer—they may be non-specific or hormonally mediated. Hyponatraemia, water retention and hypokalaemia are the commonest abnormalities. Hyponatraemia is often due to haemodilution and to gut and renal loss of sodium; hypokalaemia (with alkalosis) results from loss of potassium (particularly from wasting muscle masses) via the gut and the kidney. Renal failure from a variety of causes, exacerbates the electrolyte and acid-base problems and is often a terminal event. Dehydration (sometimes with hypernatraemia) can complicate radiotherapy and chemotherapy, particularly when gastrointestinal fluid losses are excessive in the presence of inadequate fluid intake.

Fever

Fever is common in malignant disease and particularly in lymphoreticular, kidney and hepatic neoplasms. It is however a mistake to ascribe all pyrexia to the underlying cancer, for the immunosuppression characteristic of such patients makes them more prone to infections, sometimes of occult or bizarre type.

Endocrine effects

Tumours sometimes have the capacity to secrete polypeptide hormones which are not normally secreted by the tissue from which the tumour originates; this is ectopic hormone production. This capacity is presumably as a result of derepression or activation of normally inactive nuclear genetic coding in a potentially multipotent cell type. Almost any type of polypeptide hormone can be secreted by malignant tissue, and some tumours secrete more than one ectopic hormone; the commonest tumour involved is the bronchogenic oat cell carcinoma.

Adrenocortical hyperplasia

Adrenocortical hyperplasia as a result of ectopic production of corticotrophin (ACTH) was the first syndrome to be described. Classically the onset of this form of Cushing's disease is rapid; the biochemical disturbances in the syndrome occur before the clinical manifestations which may in any case be minimal. The condition remits only if the underlying tumour, usually oat cell lung carcinoma, can be treated. Symptomatic treatment by blocking steroid production with metyrapone or aminoglutethimide may help.

Hypercalcaemia

Hypercalcaemia is not uncommon in cancer. It is seen most often with breast carcinoma and may be exacerbated in this disorder by the administration of oestrogens. Hypercalcaemia with breast carcinoma, lung carcinoma and myeloma usually occurs in the presence of bony metastases. It is likely that these deposits produce a locally reactive osteoclast stimulating substance. Sometimes, however, in these tumours and in tumours of the kidney or ovary, hypercalcaemia occurs in the absence of overt bone involvement; ectopic secretion of a parathyroid-like hormone is the likely explanation in some cases though other osteolytic substances such as prostaglandins or osteoclast activating factors may also be involved.

Hypercalcaemia, particularly if of slow onset, may be asymptomatic. More rapidly developing hypercalcaemia presents with gastrointestinal disturbances (particularly anorexia, nausea, vomiting and constipation) mental confusion (with drowsiness, psychosis or even coma) or renal failure. This situation constitutes an oncological emergency (see Chapter 19).

Inappropriate diuresis

Dilutional hyponatraemia as a result of inappropriate antidiuretic hormone (ADH) secretion (the Schwartz–Bartter syndrome) occurs most commonly in bronchogenic (oat cell) carcinoma, but has also been seen with various adenocarcinomas and in Hodgkin's disease. The inappropriate secretion of ADH in the presence of normal renal function leads to water retention with a low serum sodium, increased urinary sodium excretion and a urine osmolality exceeding that of the serum. This situation may also be seen as a complication of severe chest infection or drug therapy (e.g. vincristine). In severe or terminal illness the so-called 'sick cell syndrome' resulting from cell membrane malfunction is more likely; the serum osmolality is normal in the presence of hyponatraemia.

With hyponatraemia, lethargy with nausea and vomiting are the most prominent symptoms, though coma may supervene. Urgent treatment will only occasionally be required (see Chapter 19).

Hypoglycaemia

Hypoglycaemia, with non-pancreatic tumours, is most often seen with large low-grade retroperitoneal and mediastinal sarcomas. Excessive glucose utilisation by the tumour is an unlikely explanation for the hypoglycaemia; the production of a hypoglycaemic factor, distinct from insulin, is more probable. These symptoms are of the classical hypoglycaemic type and respond to glucose administration; they may resolve completely after surgical resection of the tumour.

Hyperthyroidism

Hyperthyroidism may result from the occasional secretion of a thyroid stimulating hormone-like polypeptide, produced along with chorionic gonadotrophin from choriocarcinoma cells. Thyroid function test disturbance is more frequent than the clinical features of thyrotoxicosis.

Precocious puberty

Precocious puberty is a rare syndrome which has been reported in young boys with malignant hepatoblastoma; the tumour appears to secrete gonadotrophin-like substances.

Gynaecomastia/HPOA

Gynaecomastia may occur in men with bronchogenic carcinoma, particularly in association with clubbing of the digits, hypertrophic pulmonary osteoarthropathy (painful periostitis in the distal portion of bony extremities) and pachydermoperiostosis (overlying chronic skin changes). The cause of this syndrome is uncertain but high levels of growth hormone-like and gonadotrophin-like substances have been found. Successful treatment of the tumour may give dramatic regression of the syndrome.

Apudomas

Apudoma (Table 16.2) is a term which has been coined for a group of syndromes which are not really of the ectopic hormone production type; rather they are the overproduction by certain tumours of polypeptide and amine

Table 16.2. Apudomas.

POLYPEPTIDE HORMONES	
Pituitary adenomas	Anterior pituitary
Medullary carcinoma	Thyroid
Hyperinsulinism	
Zollinger–Ellison syndrome	
Hyperglycaemia	Pancreas
Pancreatic cholera syndrome	
AMINE HORMONES	
Carcinoid	Small gut
Phaeochromocytoma	Adrenal medulla, sympathetic ganglia
MULTIPLE ENDOCRINE ADENOMATOSIS	Multiple

hormones appropriate to the tissue of origin of that tumour. Apudomas produce hormones of the APUD (amine content and/or amine precursor uptake and decarboxylation) type. They arise from cells originating from the ancestral neural crest and it is possible that many, if not all, of the paraneoplastic endocrine syndromes discussed above may prove to be of APUD cell origin.

Polypeptide hormones

Many apudomas secrete excessive amounts of polypeptide hormones.

Pituitary adenomas. Tumours (usually adenomas) of the basophil or chromophobe cells of the anterior pituitary, with excessive production of adrenocorticotrophic hormone, give rise to the classical Cushing's syndrome. Melanocyte stimulating hormone may also be hypersecreted, particularly after adrenalectomy for Cushing's syndrome, giving the classical Nelson's syndrome with increased pigmentation in association with an expanding pituitary tumour. Cushing's disease may be alleviated by removal of the target organs (the adrenals). An expanding pituitary tumour may need to be surgically excised or ablated by radiation, usually by radioactive implantation (see also Chapter 13).

Medullary carcinoma of the parafollicular C cells of the thyroid produces excess quantities of calcitonin. The presentation of this tumour is usually as a thyroid swelling, sometimes in association with persistent diarrhoea;

hormonal manifestations as a result of hypocalcaemia are rare but there may be compensatory overproduction of parathormone. An early medullary carcinoma is curable by surgical excision; later lesions do not respond well to chemotherapy or radiotherapy.

Hyperinsulinism with consequent hypoglycaemia, results most often from a beta cell insulin-secreting tumour (insulinoma) of the islets of Langerhans in the pancreas.

The Zollinger–Ellison syndrome of chronic peptic ulceration, diarrhoea and hypokalaemia, is due to hypersecretion of gastrin usually by tumours of the alpha cells of the islets of Langerhans in the pancreas. Diagnosis is confirmed by elevated serum gastrin levels. Tumours may be multifocal and some metastasise.

Hyperglycaemia and the *pancreatic cholera syndrome* due to excess secretion of glucagon (glucagonoma) and vasoactive intestinal peptide (vipoma) respectively, also result from islet cell tumours of the pancreas.

Treatment of all the above pancreatic tumours is by surgical excision after correction of biochemical abnormalities.

Amine hormones

Other apudomas produce their effects by oversecretion of certain physiological amine hormones. The characteristic and well known carcinoid syndrome consists of episodic flushing, diarrhoea, and bronchospasm. Later in the syndrome chronic facial telangiectasia and right-sided valvular lesions with heart failure, may ensue. The syndrome occurs late in the natural history of carcinoid tumours which are of low-grade malignancy; these tumours more often present with features due to their actual presence (e.g. intestinal obstruction or bleeding).

Carcinoid tumours occur most often in the small intestine and appendix; the carcinoid syndrome is usually seen with the jejuno-ileal lesions. Elevated levels of 5-hydroxyindolacetic acid, 5-hydroxytryptamine, 5-hydroxytryptophan or histamine can be found in the syndrome. Carcinoid tumours have also been found in other gut tissues and in foregut derivatives, particularly bronchus and pancreas. They are slow growing and are best treated if possible by surgery, though treatment with hydroxy-tryptamine and histamine antagonists has been used for symptomatic relief. Radiotherapy and cytotoxic chemotherapy have not proved helpful.

Phaeochromocytomas arise from phaeochromocytes either in the adrenal medulla (where they produce mainly adrenaline) or from the sympathetic nerve ganglia (where they secrete mainly noradrenaline). Paroxysmal or sustained hypertension with associated abnormal 'fright, fight or flight' episodes are possible clinical presentations depending on the relative amounts of adrenaline and noradrenaline secreted by the tumour. Treatment is by excision after careful preoperative alpha and beta adrenergic receptor blockade.

Multiple endocrine adenomatosis

Multiple endocrine adenomatosis (pluriglandular syndromes) is the name given to a group of syndromes in which two or more APUD hormones are hypersecreted in the same patient at some time. One form, often hereditary, is characterised by multiple endocrine adenomas particularly of the pancreas and also of the parathyroid and pituitary glands. Another form is parathyroid adenomas with phaechromocytoma and medullary thyroid carcinoma.

Dermatological effects

The non-metastatic skin manifestations of cancer may be non-specific or specific.

Non-specific manifestations

Bizarre or severe infections of the skin (e.g. severe Herpes zoster or simplex) may reflect the immunosuppressed status of the patient. Pruritus, sometimes with extensive excoriation, may denote underlying malignancy; it is particularly a feature of Hodgkin's disease. Acquired icthyosis, with dry hyperkeratotic scaly skin, may herald lymphoreticular or epithelial neoplasms. Haemorrhagic skin manifestations (e.g. purpura) may be seen in association with thrombocytopenia as a result of marrow infiltration or from the effects of radiotherapy and cytotoxic chemotherapy.

Specific manifestations

More specific manifestations of malignancy are now recognised, however. Acanthosis nigricans with velvety black epidermal hyperplasia, found particularly in skin flexures, may herald adenocarcinoma, particularly of the stomach. The diagnosis of dermatomyositis, an immunological disturbance involving skin and muscle, warrants an exhaustive search for tumour.

This may originate in any tissue but particularly in the breast, gut and lung. Exfoliative erythroderma is occasionally seen with generalised non-Hodgkin's lymphoma and is a prominent feature of the Sézary syndrome (see Chapter 11). Tylosis with hypertrophy of the skin of the palms and soles may presage oesophageal carcinoma, and erythema gyratum repens, in which an erythematous eruption moves slowly over the body, is associated with breast and lung cancers. The growth of lanugo-type hair, malignant down, on the face and upper parts of the body also heralds internal malignancy.

Neurological effects

The term 'carcinomatous neuromyopathy' has been used to encompass those neurological disorders occurring in association with, but not due to metastases from, cancer, particularly bronchogenic carcinoma. The brain, spinal cord, peripheral nerves and muscles can be involved; often more than one system is affected. The discussion below does not include reference to those disorders occurring as a result of endocrine or metabolic disturbances or of those seen with the wasting process of malignant cachexia.

Brain and spinal cord disorders

The syndrome of encephalomyelitis is a multifocal disorder in which inflammatory lesions can be seen throughout the nervous system. Cerebellar degeneration with nystagmus, ataxia and dysarthria may be a prominent feature. Lesions in the cerebrum may give dementia and personality changes. Brain stem, pyramidal tract and posterior column involvement may lead to cranial nerve palsies and to various bulbar and spinal cord syndromes, for example resembling motor neurone disease.

Nerve disorders

Neuropathies are basically of two types, primary sensory and mixed peripheral; the former results from destruction of the posterior root ganglion cells, the latter from demyelination of peripheral nerves. The pattern is often mixed however.

Muscle disorders

Muscle disorders in malignancy are of three types:
1 Proximal myopathy, with proximal muscle weakness.

2 Polymyositis, with various immunological connective tissue disorders, e.g. dermatomyositis.

3 Myasthenia.

The myasthenia-myopathic syndrome of Eaton and Lambert superficially resembles classical myasthenia gravis (which is undoubtedly associated with malignant thymoma). Muscle wasting is, however, usually more severe and brain stem innervated musculature is often spared. The response to neostigmine is usually poor and the electromyographic studies characteristic.

It is recognised that remote neurological manifestations may present before the tumour becomes evident and that occasionally treatment of the tumour improves the neurological features. In most cases, however, symptomatic treatment is all that can be offered. The features may wax and wane in severity, however, and occasionally corticosteroids promote transient improvement.

Haematological effects

Anaemia

Anaemia is very common in advanced malignant disease; it may arise from haemorrhage giving a hypochromic microcytic blood picture, from bone marrow infiltration with a leucoerythroblastic picture, or from folic acid deficiency with a macrocytic picture. Often, however, the blood film is non-specific with normocytic normochromic features; in these cases certain remote effects of the malignancy seem to be toxic to the bone marrow and there is a block to the utilisation of iron stores. Anaemia can also be due to autoantibody-mediated haemolysis, particularly in certain lymphomas and leukaemias, and of course to the cytotoxic myelosuppressive effects of cancer therapy.

White cell and platelet abnormalities

The non-specific effects of cancers are also reflected in white cell and platelet abnormalities. Marked polymorphonuclear leucocytosis with the appearance in the blood of primitive and morphologically abnormal cells (the so-called 'leukaemoid' reaction) can be a feature of widespread malignancy. Lymphopenia is an unfavourable finding in untreated malignant lymphoma. Together with anaemia and thrombocytopenia, however, leucopenia is often a finding after myelotoxic therapy. Thrombocytosis is a non-specific finding with carcinoma, and thrombocytopenia is occasionally due to the formation of autoimmune platelet antibodies.

Erythrocytosis

Erythrocytosis, which is distinct from polycythaemia vera and secondary polycythaemia, is seen most often with renal tumours, particularly hypernephroma and occasionally with cerebellar haemangioblastoma and hepatoma. It is now thought to be due to production of an erythropoietic-stimulating hormone similar to erythropoietin.

Hypercoagulability

Migrating thrombophlebitis is an established association with carcinoma (particularly of pancreas, lung and gastrointestinal tract); its cause is unknown. Non-bacterial thrombotic endocarditis with large friable fibrinous valvular vegetations may also be found. Disseminated intravascular coagulation (purpura fulminans) may complicate advanced malignancy, probably as a result of the release of thromboplastic substances into the blood stream; the intravascular clotting with resultant thrombocytopenia and hypofibrinogenaemia may have fatal consequences.

Hyperviscosity

Hyperviscosity, with tendency to thrombosis or haemorrhage, usually accompanies neoplasms with associated dysproteinaemia, particularly Waldenstrom's macroglobulinaemia and multiple myeloma or where there is marked polycythaemia. Treatment of the disorder is by plasmapheresis or venesection, with attention to the underlying malignancy.

Haemorrhage

Haemorrhage in a patient with cancer can result from thrombocytopenia (e.g. from bone marrow infiltration), from lack of coagulation factors (e.g. with gross liver disease) or from the onset of disseminated intravascular coagulation.

Immunosuppression

Immunosuppression is common in patients with widespread malignancy, particularly where there is involvement of the lymphoreticular system (see Chapter 1). The use of radiotherapy and particularly cytotoxic chemotherapy may worsen the situation and a careful watch for infections in such patients is vital.

Chapter 17
Surveillance, Palliative Support and Terminal Care

Surveillance

In assessing the need for follow-up surveillance in patients after treatment three factors are important: **1** knowledge of the biology of the tumour, **2** the pros and cons of follow-up for the patient and the doctor, **3** the importance of teamwork.

1 The behaviour of many malignancies is now understood and is predictable—they may be potentially curable (e.g. children's tumours, lymphoma, uterine carcinoma etc.), usually incurable (e.g. lung, brain) or may have a very long natural history (e.g. breast, ovary).

2 In favour of follow-up is that the patient and clinician get the psychological reassurance that all is well, that the patient will hopefully be seen at an early stage of any recurrence of disease and that accurate follow-up allows accurate statistics. Against follow-up is the possibility that the patient may be anxious or uneasy about continuous follow-up, that cured patients will be followed unnecessarily, that follow-up is time consuming and that even if things do go wrong the clinician cannot always correct them.

3 The value of community services in follow-up cannot be over-emphasised. Various community staff—GPs, nurses and social workers—play an important role, particularly when they work in close liaison with the hospital oncology service.

All things considered it is usually accepted as important for a senior hospital oncologist to supervise the follow-up of patients with close communication with other hospital specialists and with the community health team. Hopefully the oncologist will know his patient well and detect slight but significant changes; each time he sees the patient a short history is taken and relevant examination done. Malignant disease is now accepted as the great mimic and any symptom or sign should be taken as relevant to the primary cancer or its treatment until proven otherwise.

The psychological aspects of follow-up are all important. Some patients will be followed unnecessarily whereas others may be well for periods from weeks to decades after therapy. Patients may not seek medical advice spontaneously but when abnormalities are found at follow-up there is a good chance that something positive can be done, possibly with further curative therapy, if not with palliative measures.

Palliation

It is generally accepted that only about 30% of patients attending an oncology centre will be cured. Therefore, most of the workload of the centre is concerned with palliation. Palliation is a term defining an intention rather than a treatment, the aim being to restore an acceptable quality of life by giving the maximum symptomatic relief by the simplest method available with the minimum upset to the patient and in the shortest time possible. Palliation is not synonymous with terminal care and may vary from simple reassurance or analgesia for pain relief to a prolonged course of treatment, irradiation or cytotoxic. Such measures may achieve either control of local disease or symptoms without prolonging life or a prolongation of life without control of the disease, the latter being of doubtful value to the patient. A combination of general and specific measures for palliation is usually necessary (Table 17.1), and in all patients the beneficial results achieved must be balanced against the harmful effects of the treatment.

Table 17.1. Palliative measures.

GENERAL
Mental welfare (morale)
Nutritional state
Control of non-specific symptoms

SPECIFIC
Surgery
Irradiation
Cytotoxic chemotherapy

General measures

Morale

The most important factor in management is to establish a good rapport with the patient and to ensure that morale is kept to the maximum; this is usually achieved by good communication. Many doctors and students find it difficult to communicate with the patient with cancer, partly because of their own pre-existing prejudices and fears and partly because they are uncertain as to how much the patient wishes or needs to know. Communication is learnt by example and by experience; each patient presents a different attitude towards his or her disease and must be assessed individually. There is often no need to inform the patient of the whole truth; he or she will be contented and relieved by a simple explanation of the disease and would be unnecessarily worried and depressed by use of words like cancer and malignancy without adequate explanation. Other patients, however, express a desire to know the full diagnosis; the oncologist must then decide, often intuitively, whether the desire is genuine or whether what the patient really wants is reassurance. Even when the whole truth is told, however, the patient must always be given some hope of help. All patients must be encouraged to ask questions, which must be answered as expertly and as non-evasively as possible by an experienced member of staff. One result of not informing patients of the accurate diagnosis is that cured patients cannot testify as to the success of treatment and consequently pre-existing attitudes as to the incurability of cancer are further reinforced.

Even when some patients are told that they have a malignant disease or cancer they will later deny the diagnosis; a repression which emphasises the guilt felt by many patients.

Patients' relatives have a most important part to play in keeping morale high; they must be fully informed of the situation and given a reasonable idea of prognosis. The clinician must, however, watch for psychological barriers developing between the patient who is unaware and the relatives who are fully aware of the diagnosis.

Nutrition

Nutritional deficiency is a common finding in patients with cancer and many factors contribute towards what may become a cachexic state (see Chapter 16). It is likely that a lack of essential foodstuffs, vitamins and minerals contributes towards the non-specific illness associated with cancer, and attempts to nourish the patient may be extremely beneficial. The presentation of an attractive supplemented diet, correction of oral disorders, treatment of nausea and vomiting, and psychological encouragement are the simplest means of enforcing adequate diet; in the extremely ill-nourished individual, however, enteral or intravenous feeding may be warranted.

Non-specific symptoms

The patient with cancer may have many non-specific problems (e.g. dermatitis, nausea, constipation, diarrhoea) some associated with the tumour, others with the treatment. As always a sympathetic ear, relevant physical examination and reassurance are usually far better than any drug. Should drug treatment be required it is better to prescribe simple tested remedies and to avoid polypharmacy.

Specific measures

Surgery

Surgery may be required among other things for removal of recurrent masses (diagnostic, therapeutic or cosmetic), relief of obstructive symptoms (as for example in the bowel), for relief of pain (e.g. by nerve section) or for the immobilisation of pathological fractures.

Irradiation

Irradiation may be needed to relieve obstruction, to control pain, to control unsightly or smelly tumour fungation, to control haemorrhage, or simply to shrink or even arrest rapidly growing obvious lesions.

Chemotherapy

Chemotherapy may give pain relief, control of fungation, control of rapidly enlarging obvious lesions and may, if locally administered, stop the reaccumulation of effusions.

Terminal care

At some stage it will be obvious to the doctor that the patient with an unresponsive cancer is terminally ill. He will have excluded remediable illness associated with the cancer and must now continue palliation without prolonging a miserable existence. At this stage there are three places in which the patient can die comfortably. If home circumstances allow and if the relatives and family doctor are willing and able to cope, then many patients with cancer express the preference to die at home. The community team has a very important role to play in this situation and the patient and his family must be given every support for their social and emotional needs. The patient may die in the oncological or general hospital where he or she has had the treatment. This may be best for the patient who shows rapid deterioration and has poor home circumstances; he or she is in constant contact with the medical and nursing staff who have been present throughout the illness. Many oncology centres now have access to specially run units (sometimes independently funded) for patients with terminal cancer; the nursing and emotional needs of the patient are particularly well cared for in such units by specially trained staff. A compromise between home and hospital care for pre-terminal patients has been developed in some areas—the cancer day hospital run as an integral part of a terminal care unit. Most patients attending such a hospital eventually die in the terminal care unit having had a period of intermediate adjustment.

Terminal features

Whenever a patient is dying certain features are prominent terminally. These are pain, nausea and vomiting, psychiatric disturbances, and respiratory, urinary and gastrointestinal problems. As always the morale of a patient is of paramount importance; he or she needs to be constantly talked to and reassured by medical and nursing staff. At this stage the patient may want to talk about dying or may need to be assured that it will not be a painful, miserable or lonely process. Great benefit is often gained by communication with members of the religious clergy.

Pain

The pain of terminal cancer is often heightened by fear of the unknown; reassurance and explanation will often result in lessening of this symptom. In cases of persistent pain it is important that analgesia is administered regularly, for example on a 4–6 hourly basis, rather than on demand by the patient. If pain is not relieved by simple analgesics (e.g. paracetamol) an intermediate potency group of drugs, including dihydrocodeine, pentazocine and dextromoramide, is available. For severe persistent pain strong narcotic drugs are mandatory; addiction is not a problem in the terminally ill patient. Diamorphine is the most satisfactory of this group; it may be combined in various Brompton-type cocktails with cocaine and/or chlorpromazine, but diamorphine alone in flavoured syrup suits many patients. A recently marketed sustained release tablet form of morphine sulphate is also proving very effective in this situation. Parenteral administration of diamorphine may be the only answer to some forms of terminal pain.

Many analgesics have adverse as well as beneficial effects. Drowsiness may be a prominent but sometimes not unwelcome effect. Nausea and constipation are sometimes troublesome.

Nausea and vomiting

Nausea and vomiting can be very distressing. If these symptoms are obstructive in origin nasogastric suction may be helpful; if non-specific or related to other essential medication anti-emetic drugs may be necessary. Metoclopramide, prochlorperazine and certain other phenothiazines can be given, if necessary by suppository or by injection. Dyspepsia is alleviated by administration of antacids.

Psychiatric disturbances

Psychiatric disturbances are common in terminal disease. Anxiety and depression are helped as much by reassurance as by medication, but severe symptoms may warrant benzodiazepine tranquilliser (e.g. diazepam) or tricyclic anti-depressant (e.g. amitriptyline) therapy. Confusion, as a non-specific effect of cancer and its complications, is helped by phenothiazine drugs or by haloperidol. Surprisingly insomnia is a common complaint in the terminally ill patient at home; nitrazepam is usually effective.

Respiratory disturbances

Respiratory disturbances include dyspnoea, often combined with anxiety, coughing and hiccups. Dyspnoea, if due to a large fluid effusion, will obviously be helped by aspiration of fluid. If due to pulmonary disease then diamorphine or diazepam, alone or in combination, given with reassurance, will prove extremely helpful. The latter therapy will also be found to be effective in troublesome coughing, though this symptom may also be controlled with a strong (e.g. methadone) linctus. Intractable hiccups usually responds to chlorpromazine.

Urinary incontinence

Urinary incontinence may be due to excess sedation, to the presence of vesical fistulae, or to urinary retention with overflow, often in association with severe constipation. Readjustment of medication, clearing of the loaded rectum or as a final resort catheterisation of the bladder may be necessary.

Constipation

Constipation is very common in terminally ill immobile patients, particularly those on strong analgesics; administration of simple laxatives or of rectal enemata may avoid the problem of spurious diarrhoea from impacted rectal faeces.

Nursing care

Throughout the terminal illness nursing care to avoid pressure sores, to give oral hygiene, to dress fungating or offensive lesions, and above all to ensure mental and bodily comfort is the mainstay of management.

Chapter 18
Education, Screening
and Prevention

Education

Fear is the main cause of delay in seeking medical advice by patients with cancer or a suspicion of having cancer. This is easily understood because many people still regard cancer as incurable and associated with great pain and suffering. Many will have had experience of relatives, friends or acquaintances with terminal cancer, and will have vivid recollections of the problems. Few will know of or remember patients cured of the disease, because usually this is less dramatic and less of a talking point in general. The supposed association of pain with cancer applies also to early disease; patients often say that they did not suspect that a lump could be malignant because it was not painful.

It is of great importance therefore to emphasise that many patients can be cured of cancer, and that if cure is not achieved high-grade palliation is often possible, and also that pain is not inevitable even in advanced disease.

Examples of the better prognosis from the treatment of early disease as compared with late disease are given in Table 18.1, in which 5-year survival rates are quoted.

Table 18.1. Prognosis in early and late cancer.

Tumour type	Early disease	Late disease
Skin (squamous)	90%	30%
Cervix uteri (squamous)	80%	3%
Larynx	90%	20%
Breast	75%	5%
Bladder	70%	5%

The use of 5-year survival figures does not represent the longer term prognosis for all malignancies, but with the exception of cancer of the breast it is a realistic indication of the probable very long-term prognosis for all the types listed in the table.

Thus, treatment of a higher proportion of cancers at an earlier stage would yield much improved results.

Another important cause of delay in seeking medical advice is genuine ignorance of the possibly serious nature of a symptom or sign. It is still thought by many that a painless lump in the breast cannot be a cancer, that irregular vaginal bleeding in middle age must be due to 'the change', that persistent hoarseness must be due to chronic laryngitis, and that a persistent ulcer of the skin must be due to 'poor healing flesh'.

Education directed towards a better understanding of the signs and symptoms of early cancer is needed. This must be planned and presented carefully, or a person who is ignorant of the early manifestations of cancer may be converted into one who is afraid of the disease.

Yet another barrier to the early diagnosis of cancer is the view still held by some people that the disease is associated with uncleanliness or immorality; some harbour a feeling of guilt about the condition. One major aim of education must be the acceptance of cancer on the same level as other diseases.

In cancer education programmes the mass media are of limited value. The presentation of facts and figures to an immense audience demands the use of dogmatic statements with little opportunity for qualifying these or elaborating upon variations and exceptions to them, and there is no facility for questions and answers.

A much more effective forum is the smaller group in the community, for example the Round Table group, the church group or the Young Mother's group. Points which are not understood can be elaborated and clarified, and above all particular questions from individuals can be answered.

Cancer education is relevant not only to the general public. Some medical practitioners, medical students, nurses, health visitors, and social workers have unduly pessimistic views about cancer and its response to treatment. Perhaps this is not entirely without foundation as inevitably many doctors and nurses are more involved with patients who cannot be treated effectively, or in whom treatment has failed.

Cancer education schemes are established in some areas, and surveys are showing that increasing numbers of people believe that some cancers can be cured, and that the earlier the diagnosis is made the better are the chances of cure.

The argument that public education about cancer will aggravate existing fears and therefore add to the delay, or will lead to the medical profession being inundated with unnecessarily anxious patients, carries little weight in practice.

On the other hand, well-conducted cancer education will be wasted or brought into disrepute if due attention is not given to the possible early symptoms and signs of the disease, or if facilities are not readily available for the investigation of patients who present in response to that education.

Education programmes cost money, but effective ones result in earlier treatment of many cancers with better responses and less subsequent expenditure on the treatment of residual, recurrent or metastatic disease or on terminal nursing care. On purely financial grounds, therefore, they are to be commended, quite apart from the reduction in the burden of suffering and distress from malignancy which may be eradicated completely were there a better appreciation of the situation by the patient.

Screening

A detectable cancer is seldom 'early' in the absolute sense; the earliest demonstrable tumour will have passed most of its natural life and may have established occult metastases.

It is difficult to detect a tumour much less than 1 cm in diameter, unless it is in an accessible site. A tumour of this size would contain about 10^9 cells. If its cell doubling time were 100 days (a realistic estimate), if this time remained constant, if the tumour arose from a single cell, and if no cells were lost during growth, the 1 cm diameter tumour would have originated about 10 years previously (i.e. 30 doubling times ago). A subsequent interval of 2½ years would lead to a tumour about 8 cm in diameter, and a further 1½ years to a mass of about half the body weight of an adult person.

Before a tumour has produced symptoms or signs the only way to detect its presence is by the routine examination of 'well' persons. Cancer screening programmes have been established for this. Initially, these programmes were directed at specific groups of people 'at risk' occupationally, for example workers in the rubber and cable industries, and aniline dye workers. Now they have been extended to cover a much wider field, including the general population in some aspects, for example cervical smears for the detection of carcinoma-in-situ.

To be effective and acceptable a cancer screening programme must satisfy certain criteria. The aim is to screen large numbers of people who otherwise would not consult a doctor or feel the need for routine checks. Therefore, publicity is important and must be sufficiently wide to reach all classes of the population.

Administration must be simple and expenses for accommodation, staff, equipment and 'expendables' must be low. The cancer detection rates will be low; for example about five cases of carcinoma-in-situ of the cervix uteri are found for every 1000 women screened over the age of 25 years, and all of these will not progress to established cancer.

The procedures involved must be completed quickly, and tests should not require hospital admission. Healthy people are likely to be reluctant to lose much time off work or household duties. The examinations must be acceptable; few people are going to submit to uncomfortable or painful procedures in the interests of possibly detecting an abnormality which is asymptomatic and for which the 'risk' of detection is about 0.5%.

The tests must be easily processed and interpreted. Complex procedures are expensive, and results which are not precise are of very limited value. The reliability of results also must be high. The ideal tests are those which yield no false positive and no false negative results; this ideal is rarely achieved in practice.

When positive results are obtained facilities must be available for the rapid referral of the person to the appropriate specialist. Equivocal or suspicious results must lead to further investigations to clarify the situation.

The need for regular repeat examinations must be stressed, and these made available at intervals appropriate to the type of test. Many people assume that screening tests are a 'once-and-for-all' procedure, not realising that with the passage of time a negative test may become positive.

Not infrequently people routinely screened for malignant disease are found to have other unrelated abnormalities of which they were unaware, or the nature of which they did not appreciate. Such findings provide an incidental bonus to routine screening procedures.

The complexity of screening tests ranges from the simple cervical smear to sophisticated investigations such as endoscopy and contrast radiography. The complexity and therefore the expense of the more involved investigations greatly limits their general applicability to screening programmes. Nevertheless they remain applicable to the detailed screening of selected groups of persons at special risk, for example those industrially exposed to carcinogens.

Other techniques available include cytological examination of gastric and colonic washings, bronchial aspirates and centrifuged deposits of urine, radiological examination of the female breast (mammography), thermography of the female breast, ultrasound scanning of the abdomen and pelvis, and the scanning of organs using radioisotopes. A recent addition to the screening armamentarium is the examination of blood samples for abnormal proteins which may be related to certain cancers—the so-called tumour markers. However, in the main such tumour markers are not specific for single tumour types or indeed for cancer itself.

The simplest of all screening procedures is that of self examination of the female breast. If undertaken properly it can reveal a mass long before it would be evident spontaneously or would be discovered by chance, and should therefore show a better prognosis from treatment.

Again, education is an essential prerequisite for any successful screening programme.

Prevention

As epidemiological studies progress it is becoming increasingly apparent that many cancers are due to carcinogens, not only of occupational origin, but also present in the general environment to which all people are exposed.

Reference has been made to known carcinogenic factors in certain occupations (see Chapter 1). Once a carcinogen is identified steps can be taken to prevent exposure to it, by careful screening or handling techniques, or by substituting a non-carcinogenic agent.

In the environment at large identification of carcinogens or potential carcinogens is much more difficult. Atmospheric pollution associated with industrial conditions must be an important source of such agents.

Chemicals used as pesticides, fertilisers, preservatives, and colouring and flavouring agents may have carcinogenic properties. Food cooking and treatment processes, for example smoke-curing of fish, may produce carcinogenic substances in the food.

The types of food in the diet, and the absence of certain vitamins may be factors in carcinogenesis. The incidence of cancer of the upper alimentary tract, for example, can be related in part to chronic alcoholism.

Study of the chemical structure of known carcinogens may provide a lead to the possible carcinogenicity of other substances. However, to prove or disprove this may take a long time, because of the long latent periods of action of most carcinogens.

In some malignancies hygienic factors are important, the best recognised being poor dental hygiene and malignancy in the buccal cavity, and poor hygiene in relation to cancer of the penis and uterine cervix.

The control of environmental carcinogens may seem easy in theory, but can be difficult in practice. Control may require radical changes in social and dietary habits, or even exclusion of some time-honoured processes, foods, drinks or habits. Much might be achieved by education; some factors need legislation for their control.

Chapter 19
Oncological Emergencies

Superior vena cava obstruction

The syndrome of superior vena cava obstruction usually results from pressure on the superior vena cava by tumour masses in the superior mediastinum; occasionally, it is due to actual tumour involvement of the vessel and mural thrombus formation. The commonest cause is lymph node metastases from a primary carcinoma of the bronchus. It is much less common from node enlargement by lymphoma, or from thymoma or other mediastinal tumours. Development of the syndrome may be gradual or rapid; in the latter case, superimposed thrombosis is the likely cause.

Classically, there is over-filling and distention of the veins of the head, neck and upper limbs, and dilated subcutaneous veins over the front of the chest and of the abdomen, the latter being a manifestation of colateral circulation to the inferior vena cava. There is associated oedema of the tissues, and in severe cases suffusion of the conjunctivae.

Initial responses to radiation or chemotherapy are often good. It is an observed fact that only partial regression of the mediastinal mass can lead to complete regression of the signs of obstruction. Thrombosis of the superior vena cava will not respond to irradiation; also, it seldom responds to anti-coagulant therapy. When radiotherapy is the method of choice this should be fractionated; in severe cases, the dose for the first exposure may be increased with the aim of gaining a more rapid response.

Development of superior vena cava obstruction from bronchial carcinoma carries a bad prognosis; the average survival being of the order of 4–6 months.

Progressive obstruction to the main bronchi or lower trachea with stridor also presents an emergency situation. Rapid symptomatic improvement usually follows radiation therapy, especially for undifferentiated small cell carcinoma of the bronchus. For sensitive tumours, cytotoxic chemotherapy may be equally effective. In the acute phase, dexamethasone may also be helpful.

Spinal cord compression

Evidence of spinal cord compression may indicate a surgical emergency. Pressure from tumour masses within the spinal canal, or from vertebral body collapse from metastatic involvement, will lead to local ischaemia and to degeneration of nerve fibres if this is severe or prolonged. Degeneration of non-myelinated fibres within the cord is permanent and recovery does not occur. Partial ischaemia, however, is compatible with some degree of recovery of function if the pressure is relieved. Therefore, decompression is indicated as quickly as possible.

If the lesion is a primary one, surgical decompressive laminectomy must be considered, especially if this can be undertaken within 48 hours of development of the condition.

Secondary tumour deposits present a less well-defined situation. If the prognosis for the primary tumour is not bad, and the deposit appears to be solitary, laminectomy is to be recommended. On the other hand, the presence of multiple bony lesions in the spine or of extensive bone destruction locally, may argue against surgical intervention. In such cases, dexamethasone therapy may be of value in limiting reactive oedema, and local palliative radiation therapy will usually reduce associated pain and may produce sufficient tumour regression to allow some recovery of function. The use of high-energy radiation has the advantage of producing less skin reaction, and this may be of great benefit for patients requiring prolonged nursing in bed.

Cytotoxic chemotherapy may be of limited value, but only for very sensitive tumours, such as undifferentiated small cell carcinoma of the bronchus, or lymphoma if this is extradural, or in situations where there is not immediate access to surgery or radiation therapy.

Altered consciousness

As in any branch of medicine, coma of apparently unknown cause is a not uncommon problem in oncology. It is important not to jump to the immediate conclusion that altered consciousness (varying from drowsiness or confusion, to full blown coma) is due to some manifestation of the cancer. The 'pressure' effects of secondary deposits may be responsible, but it is important to exclude other potentially remediable causes.

Status epilepticus resulting from cerebral secondary deposits can lead to profound coma; good recovery is possible with appropriate anti-convulsant therapy.

Drug overdose (deliberate or iatrogenic) is a particular problem where strong opiate analgesics are being used. A history of escalating doses to combat increasing pain or of anxiety/depression and suicidal thoughts may be obtained; constricted pupils are an additional clue. This situation responds dramatically to intravenous naloxone, an opiate antagonist.

Acute, and less often chronic, e.g. tuberculous, infection may cause
diagnostic difficulties—toxic confusional states are not uncommon; pyrexia
is usually present to aid diagnosis.

Metabolic disturbance, as a manifestation of the cancer or its treatment,
is often reversible. A watch for hyperglycaemia is vital where steroids are
used. Hypercalcaemia and hyponatraemia, particularly when acute or
rapidly progressive, can cause bizarre cerebral features culminating in
coma.

Cerebral vascular accidents may occur coincidentally or as a complication of associated haematological abnormalities (e.g. thrombocytopenia).

Hypercalcaemia

Hypercalcaemia may be a feature of many cancers, and as we have seen
is not necessarily associated with overt bone involvement. If slow in
onset it may be asymptomatic; more rapidly developing hypercalcaemia
presents with gastrointestinal disturbances (particularly anorexia, nausea,
vomiting and constipation), mental confusion (with drowsiness, psychosis
or even coma) or renal failure. In the acute management of hypercalcaemia
rehydration is of paramount importance together with efforts to treat the
underlying cancer. If rehydration alone is not successful other measures
which may be used include the administration of oral or intravenous
phosphate, though this may achieve a reduction in plasma calcium at the
expense of precipitating calcium phosphate in the tissues (particularly the
kidneys, thus further impairing renal function). Agents which inhibit
mobilization of calcium may be required (e.g. mithramycin, corticosteroids
or calcitonin). The first of these is myelotoxic and cannot be given for
more than a few days. The latter two therapies may be successful in slowly
reducing the calcium level but may be totally ineffective even in large
doses. Recent results with diphosphonates, which act by reducing calcium
turnover, are extremely promising; these agents may establish their place
in the first-line treatment of severe or persistent hypercalcaemia when
rehydration is not effective. They can be used to keep the calcium level
down while appropriate anti-cancer treatment is initiated.

Hyponatraemia

Hyponatraemia *per se* is not uncommon (see Chapter 16). It only rarely requires urgent correction, though in its more florid forms therapy consists of
restriction of fluid intake together with the administration of demeclocycline
(a tetracycline believed to act by blocking the renal tubular effect of antidiuretic hormone) or the administration of sodium chloride, either by mouth

or by saline infusion. Treatment of the underlying neoplasm, if possible, is of paramount importance.

Infection

As we have seen, patients with cancer, particularly those involving the lymphoreticular and haematological systems may have defects in immunity and these may be exaggerated by the effects of radio- and chemotherapy. Consequently infections of various sorts are a constant source of worry.

One common problem encountered in oncology is the patient with pyrexia. This can rarely be a feature of the tumour itself (e.g. Hodgkin's disease and renal carcinoma). It is seldom the result of tumour necrosis after treatment; much more often it is a direct consequence of infection, particularly in patients who are myelosuppressed as a result of therapy. The infection may be ill-localized and pyrexia the only outward sign apart from the patient being ill. Any infective agent may cause pyrexia but it is often a common pathogen which is the offender.

Septicaemia is an oncological emergency; it has a high mortality rate and is easily missed or the diagnosis delayed. The policy must be to culture whatever specimen is available (perhaps most importantly the blood) and to get on with treatment with broad spectrum antibiotics. Bacteria most commonly encountered are *Escherichia coli*, streptococci, *Staphylococcus aureus*, and other Gram-positive organisms. There are numerous well-tested antibiotic combinations to use in this situation; our own policy is to combine piperacillin with gentamicin and to continue treatment for 5 days after the cessation of pyrexia. Viral infections such as Herpes simplex and Herpes zoster/Varicella (particularly when severe) warrant the use of intravenous acyclovir. With fungal infections anti-fungal agents such as amphotericin must be given, if necessary systemically. With Pneumocystis high-dose co-trimoxazole is usually effective.

Further Reading

General textbooks

Comprehensive reference books covering all aspects of cancer.

De Vita, V.T., Hellman, S. & Rosenberg, S.A. (1985) *Cancer, Principles and Practice of Oncology*, 2nd Edition. Lippincott, Philadelphia.
del Regato, J.A., Spjut, H.J. & Cox, J.D. (1985) *Ackerman and del Regato's Cancer Diagnosis, Treatment and Prognosis*, 6th Edition. Mosby, St Louis.
Halnan, K.E. (1982) *Treatment of Cancer*. Chapman & Hall, London.

Radiotherapy

Easson, E.C. & Pointon, R.C.S. (1985) *The Radiotherapy of Malignant Disease*. Springer-Verlag, Berlin. (A good general textbook of radiotherapy, based on the practice of the Christie Hospital and Holt Radium Institute.)
Fletcher, G.H. (1980) *Textbook of Radiotherapy*, 3rd Edition. Lea & Febiger, Philadelphia. (An authoritative American textbook of radiotherapy.)
Moss, W.T., Battifora, H. & Brand, W.N. (1979) *Radiation Oncology: Rationale, Technique and Results*, 5th Edition. Mosby, St Louis. (Therapeutic radiology in all its applications.)
Walter, J., Miller, H. & Bomford, C.K. (1979) *A Short Text-book of Radiotherapy*, 4th Edition. Churchill Livingstone, Edinburgh. (Written mainly for radiographers, but well written and comprehensive in its coverage.)

Cancer medicine

Bagshawe, K.D. (1975) *Medical Oncology*. Blackwell Scientific Publications, Oxford. (An authoritative, well informed review of the medical aspects of malignant disease.)

Calman, K.C. & Paul, R. (1978) *An Introduction to Cancer Medicine.* Macmillan, London. (A good introduction to basic scientific and clinical principles.)

Green, J.A., Macbeth, F.R., Williams, C.J. & Whitehouse, J.M.A. (1983) *Medical Oncology (Pocket Consultant).* Blackwell Scientific Publications, Oxford. (Concise practical guide to management problems in cancer medicine.)

Pinedo, H.M. & Chabner, B.A. *Cancer Chemotherapy: The EORTC Cancer Chemotherapy Annual.* Elsevier, Amsterdam. (Up-to-date, well referenced articles on current chemotherapy trends.)

Priestman, T.J. (1980) *Cancer Chemotherapy: An Introduction*, 2nd Edition. Farmitalia Carlo Erba, London. (An excellent easy-to-read introduction to clinical cancer chemotherapy.)

Index